first place
4health
Bible Study Series

a new
beginning

Christin Ditchfield

Published by Gospel Light
Ventura, California, U.S.A.
www.gospellight.com
Printed in the U.S.A.

Caution: The information contained in this book is intended to be solely for
informational and educational purposes. It is assumed that the First Place 4 Health
participant will consult a medical or health professional before beginning this or
any other weight-loss or physical fitness program.

Library of Congress Cataloging-in-Publication Data
A new beginning.
p. cm. — (First place 4 health Bible study series)
ISBN 978-0-8307-5729-9 (trade paper)
1. Christian life—Biblical teaching—Textbooks. 2. Health—Religious
aspects—Christianity.
BS680.C47N49 2011
248.4—dc22
2010043016

Rights for publishing this book outside the U.S.A. or in non-English
languages are administered by Gospel Light Worldwide, an international
not-for-profit ministry. For additional information, please visit
www.glww.org, email info@glww.org, or write to Gospel Light Worldwide,
1957 Eastman Avenue, Ventura, CA 93003, U.S.A.

To order copies of this book and other Gospel Light products in bulk
quantities, please contact us at 1-800-446-7735.

contents

BIBLE STUDIES

ADDITIONAL MATERIALS

about the author

Christin Ditchfield is host of the internationally syndicated radio program *Take It to Heart!*® Using real-life stories, rich word pictures, biblical illustrations and touches of humor, she calls believers to enthusiastically seek after God, giving them practical tools to help deepen their personal relationship with Christ. Christin is an accomplished educator, popular conference speaker and author of more than 60 books, including *A Family Guide to the Bible* and *A Way with Words: What Women Should Know About the Power They Possess.* She holds a Masters' Degree in biblical theology from Southwestern University. For more information about Christin and her ministry, visit her website at www.TakeItToHeartRadio.com.

foreword

My introduction to Bible study came when I joined First Place in March 1981. I had been attending church since I was a small child, but the extent of my study of the Bible had been reading my Sunday School quarterly on Saturday night. On Sunday morning, I would listen to my Sunday School teacher as she taught God's Word to me. During the worship service, I would listen to our pastor as he taught God's Word to me. Frankly, the idea of digging out the truths of the Bible for myself had never entered my mind.

Perhaps you are right where I was back in 1981. If so, you are in for a blessing you never dreamed possible. As you start studying the truths of the Bible for yourself through the First Place 4 Health Bible studies, you will see God begin to open your understanding of His Word.

Almost every First Place 4 Health member I have talked with about the program says, "The weight loss is wonderful, but the most important thing I have received from my association with First Place 4 Health is learning to study God's Word." The First Place 4 Health Bible studies are designed to be done on a daily basis. As you work through each day's study (which will take 15 to 20 minutes to complete), you will be discovering the deep truths of God's Word. A part of each week's study will also include a Bible memory verse for the week.

There are many in-depth Bible studies on the market. The First Place 4 Health Bible studies are not designed for the purpose of in-depth study, but are designed to be used in conjunction with the rest of the program to bring balance into your life. Our desire is for each member to begin having a personal quiet time with God each day. This time alone with God should include a time of prayer, Bible reading and Bible study. Having a quiet time is a daily discipline that will bring the rich rewards of balance, which is something we all need.

God bless you as you begin this exciting journey toward a balanced life. God will richly bless your efforts to give Him first place in your life. Remember Matthew 6:33: "But seek first his kingdom and his righteousness, and all these things will be given to you as well."

Carole Lewis, First Place 4 Health National Director

introduction

First Place 4 Health is a Christ-centered health program that emphasizes balance in the physical, mental, emotional and spiritual areas of life. The First Place 4 Health program is meant to be a daily process. As we learn to keep Christ first in our lives, we will find that He is the One who satisfies our hunger and our every need.

This Bible study is designed to be used in conjunction with the First Place 4 Health program but can be beneficial for anyone interested in obtaining a balanced lifestyle. The Bible study has been created in a five-day format, with the last two days reserved for reflection on the material studied. Keep in mind that the ultimate goal of studying the Bible is not only for knowledge but also for application and a changed life. Don't feel anxious if you can't seem to find the *correct* answer. Many times, the Word will speak differently to different people, depending on where they are in their walk with God and the season of life they are experiencing. Be prepared to discuss with your fellow First Place 4 Health members what you learned that week through your study.

There are some additional components included with this study that will be helpful as you pursue the goal of giving Christ first place in every area of your life:

- **Group Prayer Request Form:** This form is at the end of each week's study. You can use this to record any special requests that might be given in class.

- **Leader Discussion Guide:** This discussion guide is provided to help the First Place 4 Health leader guide a group through this Bible study. It includes ideas for facilitating a First Place 4 Health class discussion for each week of the Bible study.

- **Two Weeks of Menu Plans with Recipes:** There are 14 days of meals, and all are interchangeable. Each day totals 1,400 to 1,500 calories and includes snacks. Instructions are given for those who need more calories. An accompanying grocery list includes items needed for each week of meals.

- **First Place 4 Health Member Survey:** Fill this out and bring it to your first meeting. This information will help your leader know your interests and talents.

- **Personal Weight and Measurement Record:** Use this form to keep a record of your weight loss. Record any loss or gain on the chart after the weigh-in at each week's meeting.

- **Weekly Prayer Partner Forms:** Fill out this form before class and place it into a basket during the class meeting. After class, you will draw out a prayer request form, and this will be your prayer partner for the week. Try to call or email the person sometime before the next class meeting to encourage that person.

- **Live It Trackers:** Your Live It Tracker is to be completed at home and turned in to your leader at your weekly First Place 4 Health meeting. The Tracker is designed to help you practice mindfulness and stay accountable with regard to your eating and exercise habits. Step-by-step instructions for how to use the Live It Tracker are provided in the *Member's Guide*.

- **Let's Count Our Miles!** A worthy goal we encourage is for you to complete 100 miles of exercise during your 12 weeks in First Place 4 Health. There are many activities listed on pages 255-256 that count toward your goal of 100 miles. When you complete a mile of activity, mark off the box listed on the Hundred Mile Club chart located on the inside of the back cover.

- **Scripture Memory Cards:** These cards have been designed so you can use them while exercising. It is suggested that you punch a hole in the upper left corner and place the cards on a ring. You may want to take the cards in the car or to work so you can practice each week's Scripture memory verse throughout the day.

- **Scripture Memory CD:** All 10 Scripture memory verses have been put to music at an exercise tempo in the CD at the back of this study. Use this CD when exercising or even when you are just driving in your car. The words of Scripture are often easier to memorize when accompanied by music.

welcome to
A New Beginning

At your first group meeting for this session of First Place 4 Health, you will meet your fellow members, get an overview of your materials and find out what you can expect at weekly meetings. The majority of your class time will be spent learning about the four-sided person concept, the Live It Food Plan, and how change begins from the inside out. You will also have a chance to ask any questions about how to get the most out of First Place 4 Health. If possible, complete the Member Survey on page 205 before your first group meeting. The information that you give will help your leader tailor the next 12 weeks to the needs of the whole group.

Each weekly meeting begins with a weigh-in for members. This will allow you to track your progress over the 12-week session. Your Week One weigh-in/measurement will establish a baseline of comparison so that you can set healthy goals for this session. If you are apprehensive about weighing in every week, talk with your group leader about your concerns. He or she will have some options for you to consider that will make the weigh-in activity encouraging rather than stressful.

The day after your first meeting, begin Week Two of this Bible study. This session, you and your group will explore 10 key scriptural principles that will help you renew your commitment to live the life God has called you to—a life of obedience, a life of balance, a life of victory! As you open yourself to the truth of Scripture and share your hopes and struggles with the members of your group during the next 12 weeks, you'll find yourself becoming the healthy child of God you are designed to be!

making a
fresh start

SCRIPTURE MEMORY VERSE
*Therefore, if anyone is in Christ, he is a new creation;
the old has gone, the new has come!*
2 CORINTHIANS 5:17

Have you ever started a brand-new year—or a new season—full of good intentions, ready to make some serious lifestyle changes, only to see all of your resolutions fall by the wayside, one by one? Maybe your resolve lasted a few hours, a few days, a few weeks. But despite your best efforts, a series of unexpected interruptions, distractions, temptations or crises derailed your progress. Frustration led to discouragement, maybe even despair.

The good news is that God is the God of second chances, fresh starts and new beginnings! You don't have to let another day—let alone another year—go by before you start again on the path of obedience, the path that leads to balance in every area of your life, the path that leads to victory! Perhaps you've begun to experience this victory already. Maybe you've already made significant progress in some important areas of your life. But you know you haven't arrived yet—you still have a long way to go. You want to stay standing strong and not let your hard-won victory slip from your grasp.

The apostle Paul knew he hadn't arrived yet either. He compared a life of faith to running in a race, one that takes a lifetime to complete: "Forgetting what is behind and straining toward what is ahead, I press on toward the goal to win the prize for which God has called me heavenward in Christ Jesus" (Philippians 3:13-14).

God's Word tells us that God wants us to get past our failures and mistakes—to get past the guilt, past the discouragement, past the despair. He also wants us to get past the complacency that sometimes follows success—past the assumption that we know the way He will lead us, past the expectation that He will work in our hearts and lives the same way He did before. As God told Isaiah, "Forget the former things; do not dwell on the past. See, I am doing a new thing!" (Isaiah 43:18-19).

At the same time, the Bible tells us not to forget the *lessons* we've learned on our journey so far (see Deuteronomy 4:9; Philippians 4:9). We need to remember what God has taught us and how far He has brought us. This will free us to focus on living in the present, leaning on Jesus and looking ahead to the reward He has promised to those who persevere. When we give God our very best, He gives us His best in return. When we let Him lead, the journey becomes a grand adventure. Along the way we find courage to face the challenges and overcome the obstacles in our way. We learn not only to stand strong but also to soar in the strength of the Spirit.

God offers us a fresh start—a new beginning—each and every day. Are you ready to take Him up on it?

Day 1 — OUR CREATION

Dear God, thank You for fresh starts and new beginnings. Please take me by the hand. Guide me and strengthen me with each step I take. Amen.

This week's memory verse reminds us that if we have put our faith in Jesus, we have been made new—from the inside out! We've been given a new heart, a new mind, a new spirit. Read John 3:1-3. How did Jesus describe this transformation?

_____

_____

_____

_____

Why is this transformation necessary (see Romans 3:23)?

_____

_____

_____

_____

The Bible tells us that we're all born with a sinful nature that causes us to rebel against our Creator and violate the boundaries He has set for us, breaking the rules that He put in place to protect us and provide for us. God calls this sin. Since nothing sinful (imperfect or impure or unholy) can exist in the presence of God, our sin leads not just to physical death but also to spiritual death—eternal separation from Him. Read Romans 6:23. What priceless gift does God offer us?

_____

_____

_____

_____

According to Romans 5:6-8, who paid the penalty for our sin? Who took the punishment in our place?

_____

_____

_____

_____

When did this happen? What were we like when it occurred (see verse 6)?

_____

_____

_____

_____

Read John 3:16. What did our reconciliation—our salvation—cost God? Why was He willing to pay this price?

_____

_____

_____

_____

_____

Thanks to Jesus, we're no longer spiritually empty and starving. Charles Spurgeon, the well-known British preacher, once said, "Oh, travel-weary pilgrims in this wilderness of sin, you will never find even a morsel to satisfy the hunger of your spirit unless you find it in Christ! He is the source of peace for our life and all true joy comes from Him, and in times of trouble His presence is our comfort. There is nothing worth living for but Him, and His loving-kindness is better than life!"[1]

We don't live in guilt and condemnation. We've been forgiven, saved and set free (see John 3:17; Romans 8:1-2). Take a moment to remember when this precious truth first became a reality for you. How did it happen? When? Why did you decide to open your heart to Jesus? Share what it has meant to you and how your life is different now.

_____

_____

_____

_____

_____

If you have not yet experienced what it means to be born again, please take this moment to invite Jesus into your heart and life today (see Romans 10:9-10,13). Put your faith in Him and let His love transform you. Your life will never be the same!

Thank You, Jesus, for loving me so much that You couldn't leave me lost in sin. Let the life I live today be a reflection of my love for You. Amen.

OUR CALLING

Lord, my life belongs to You. Help me to find Your plan and Your purpose for me. In Jesus' name, amen.

Read Ephesians 2:8-10. According to this passage, we are saved through faith and not works. In other words, there is nothing we can do to earn our salvation—it is the gift of God. However, once we have been saved, what does Paul say we are to do?

_____

_____

_____

_____

Look up 1 Peter 2:9. How does this verse describe us as believers?

_____

_____

_____

To what task—what privilege and responsibility—has He called us?

_____

_____

_____

_____

The Bible teaches us that God has a special plan for our lives, a specific purpose for each one of us (see Psalm 139:13-16). He wants to do great things in us and through us! Read Jeremiah 29:11-13. What is God's plan for us (see verse 11)?

_____

_____

_____

_____

What kind of relationship does God want to have with us (see verses 12-13)?

_____

_____

_____

Read John 15:14-16. How did Jesus describe our relationship with Him?

_____

_____

_____

According to verse 16, what did Jesus call us to do?

_____

_____

_____

How can we fulfill what Jesus called us to do (see Colossians 1:10-12)?

_____

_____

_____

Lord, open my eyes. Give me a greater vision and a deeper understanding of this life You have called me to. Help me see what You see in me. Amen.

Day 3 — OUR RESPONSIBILITY

Jesus, thank You for rescuing me from the dominion of darkness, bringing me into Your kingdom of light. I praise You with my whole heart today. Amen.

Read Ephesians 5:1-4. What should characterize our new way of life, and whose example do we have to follow?

_____

_____

_____

_____

According to Ephesians 5:8-10, what responsibility do we have as "children of light"?

_____

_____

_____

Where can we find what we need to help us with this (see Psalm 119:105)?

_____

_____

_____

Now read Colossians 2:6-7 and Colossians 3:16. What are some of the ways we can become "rooted," or "grounded," in our faith?

_____

_____

_____

Studying the Bible and memorizing Scripture will help us to live out our faith. As Rich Mullins noted, "What we make of the Bible will never be as great as what the Bible will—if we let it—make of us."[2] What responsibility do we have, according to 1 Corinthians 6:19-20? Why?

_____

_____

_____

_____

How might this perspective affect your inspiration, your motivation and/or your determination to make healthier lifestyle choices?

_____

_____

_____

_____

How can the First Place 4 Health program help you honor God this way?

_____

_____

_____

_____

Lord, help me to remember the price You paid for my freedom and to honor You with the choices I make each day. In Jesus' precious name, amen.

Day 4 | GOD'S PROCESS

Dear God, please fill my heart with the joy of Your salvation. My hope is in You! Amen.

Although we have become new creations in Christ, every day we face the temptation to return to our old habits, our old way of thinking, our old way of life. The reality is that we still struggle with our old nature, even though it's been "put to death" (Romans 8:13). Read Luke 9:23. What did Jesus say His followers must do? How often must they do this?

_____

_____

_____

_____

Why is this? Because, as Scripture teaches, our salvation is both instantaneous and ongoing. Some theologians like to use the word "salvation" to refer to what happens in the moment in which we first believe and words like "sanctification" or "regeneration" to describe the ongoing process by which we become who God means us to be.

Others say it helps to think of our salvation as occurring in three tenses: past, present and future.[3] *We have been saved* by what Jesus did on the cross nearly 2,000 years ago (past). *We are being saved* as we respond to the work of the Holy Spirit in our hearts and lives today (present).

And *we will be saved* when we go to heaven (future). Or, as a wise old saint once put it, "I ain't what I want to be. I ain't what I'm gonna be. But praise God, I ain't what I used to be!" Look up Philippians 2:12. What does the apostle Paul urge us to do?

Note that in this context, "fear and trembling" does not mean being anxious or worried about our salvation. It means being reverent and being diligent to do what God asks of us. This is something to take seriously! Read James 2:14-18. What should always accompany faith?

We don't earn our salvation through good works (see Ephesians 2:8-9). But we prove that we are saved by doing good works—by learning and growing and maturing in the exercise of our faith. Turn to 2 Peter 1:3-8. According to verse 3, what has God given us?

According to verses 5-8, what characteristics should we exhibit, and why? (There are at least seven.)

1. _____
2. _____
3. _____

4. _____

5. _____

6. _____

7. _____

Read Philippians 2:13. Where do we get the desire, the motivation, the determination and the strength to resist our old nature (our flesh) and walk in our new nature (our spirit)?

_____

_____

_____

_____

Author and Bible teacher Gracie Malone put it this way: "While we are working things from the outside in, God works from the inside out. . . . He is working on our will, changing our hearts, motivating us from within; then, when we come to a place where we want what He wants, He gives us the ability to do it."[4] Turn to Hebrews 12:1-3. How does this passage describe Jesus?

_____

_____

_____

_____

As Christian preacher and Bible teacher Oswald Chambers wrote in *My Utmost for His Highest*, "Thank God for the glorious and majestic truth that His Spirit can work the very nature of Jesus into us, if we will only obey Him!"[5]

Thank You, God, that You always finish what You start. I can't wait to see the work You will do in me as I continually surrender my heart and my life to You. Amen.

OUR PROGRESS

Dear God, sometimes the road ahead seems long and the way uncertain. But I know You'll be with me—before me, behind me, beside me. Strengthen my heart today. Amen.

As believers, we are growing day by day in God's grace—learning more and more about living the kind of life that pleases Him. Read Titus 2:11-14. To what does the grace of God teach us to say no? Give some examples.

_____

_____

_____

_____

To what do we say yes? Give some examples.

_____

_____

_____

_____

All the while, what are we eagerly anticipating?

_____

_____

_____

_____

On that day, we will be done with our sin nature, once and for all. The ultimate victory will be ours! Until then, we have to remember who we are and what we're fighting for. Read 1 Peter 2:11-12. What is our relationship to the fallen (unsaved) world? What does this mean?

_____

_____

_____

_____

How does our obedience benefit the unsaved world?

_____

_____

_____

_____

Our primary motive for obedience is to bless the heart of God—to express our love for Him. Of course, obedience also benefits us. It protects us from the natural (and often painful) consequences of disobedience. According to Philippians 2:14-16, what are other benefits of our obedience?

_____

_____

_____

_____

Look up Colossians 1:21-23. How does God see us?

_____

_____

_____

_____

What did God do to make this possible (see verse 22)? What must we do (see verse 23)?

_____

_____

_____

_____

Sometimes we realize that if we're going to honor God in every area of our lives, we need to make some significant changes in how we live. This may seem overwhelming at times. Carole Lewis, national director of First Place 4 Health, has some great advice: "Start right where you are. That means taking whatever positive step is right in front of you; or in other words, 'do the next right thing.' "[6] Today, think about what is the next positive step—"the next right thing"—for you to do.

Lord, I want to do "the next right thing"—and the next one, and the next one after that. Help me see clearly and respond willingly. Amen.

REFLECTION AND APPLICATION

Day 6

Father, show me where I need balance in my life—specific areas in which I need to learn and grow. Teach me to be more and more like Jesus. Amen.

This week's memory verse, 2 Corinthians 5:17, assures us that through our faith in Jesus, we are restored and created anew. In what ways do you feel restored and created anew?

_____

_____

_____

_____

Prayerfully consider what God's goals for you might be, and ask Him to help you set a particular goal for your emotional health, spiritual health, mental health and physical health. (Note that you may have more than one goal for each area, but try to keep these goals as simple and focused as possible. Think about the next 11 weeks only!) Write these goals below.

Emotional health

_____

_____

_____

Spiritual health

_____

_____

_____

Mental health

_____

_____

_____

Physical health

_____

_____

_____

Someone once said, "God gives us dreams a size too big so that we can grow into them!" We know He will do His part—He will accomplish those things in our hearts and lives that only He can do. It's up to us to do our part—to put in the time and effort, make good choices, and develop the discipline and determination we need to succeed. Even in these things, God promises to help us—if we ask Him. List one specific step you can take toward achieving each of your goals.

_____

_____

_____

_____

_____

Looking over these goals, you may feel motivated, energized and inspired. You may also feel some anxiety, worry or fear that you won't be able to achieve them. Read each of the following verses and jot down any encouragement you receive:

Philippians 1:6

_____

_____

_____

_____

Philippians 4:13

_____

_____

_____

2 Timothy 1:7

_____

_____

_____

What Winston Churchill once said holds true for us today: "Success is not final, failure is not fatal: it is the courage to continue that counts."[7]

Lord, help me to walk in obedience to what You have shown me this week.
Give me strength to keep walking with You, day by day. Amen.

REFLECTION AND APPLICATION

Day 7

Thank You, Father, that Your love for us never ceases. Your mercies never come to an end. They are new every morning. Great is Your faithfulness! Amen.

Many of us have tried to make significant life changes before—tried to stand strong, only to stumble and fall. The more promises we've made to God, to ourselves and to others, the more guilt we have felt about having broken them. Sometimes our unhealthy choices are themselves a response to guilt we still feel about other sins.

As Christians, we know that God has forgiven our sins, but for some reason we're tempted to keep fishing them up. We relive the embarrassment and humiliation over and over again. It's a very effective form of self-sabotage! We end up staggering along in our Christian walk, weighed down by shame and regret. Yet 1 John 1:9 clearly tells us that "if we confess our sins, he is faithful and just and will forgive us our sins and purify us from all unrighteousness." This is a truth we need to take to heart today.

Our enemy, the devil, tries to keep us in bondage to the sins of our past. The father of lies wants to fill us with guilt and despair. But this is one time when we've got to forget our feelings and focus on the facts, as we read them in God's Word. The Bible says the blood of Jesus was shed for us. His blood cleanses us from all our sin. We've been forgiven. We've been set free. And He whom the Son has set free is "free indeed" (John 8:36)! Christian author and speaker (and Nazi holocaust survivor) Corrie ten Boom was fond of quoting Micah 7:19, which declares that God has "cast all our sins into the depths of the sea" (*NKJV*). Often she would add that He has put up a sign that reads "No Fishing."

So when you find past sins and failures flashing through your mind, resist the urge to relive them—and don't go fishing! Instead, praise God for His amazing grace. Thank Him that He really has forgiven you—whether you "feel" forgiven or not. Memorize a Scripture you can repeat to yourself whenever the memories come back to haunt you. This week's memory verse is a great one to start with, and you should by now have it memorized (for practice, say it aloud right now). Follow this one with the other Scripture verses you'll learn over the next weeks. And of course, feel free to memorize any other verses that speak to you personally.

Decide that this week, you will stand strong by standing on God's Word and make the most of this new beginning, this fresh start, this new creation—you!

Lord Jesus, it's in Your forgiveness I trust, it's in Your love that I rest, it's in Your righteousness and by Your grace that I stand. Hallelujah! Amen.

Notes
1. Charles Spurgeon, quoted in Jim Reimann, *Look Unto Me: The Devotions of Charles Spurgeon* (Grand Rapids, MI: Zondervan, 2008), p. 223.
2. Rich Mullins, *The World as I Remember It: Through the Eyes of a Ragamuffin* (Sisters, OR: Multnomah, 2004), p. 48.
3. Herbert Lockyer, Sr., gen. ed., *The Illustrated Dictionary of the Bible* (Nashville, TN: Thomas Nelson, 1986), p. 939.

4. Gracie Malone, *LifeOvers: Upside-Down Ways to Become More Like Jesus* (Grand Rapids, MI: Fleming H. Revell, 2007), p. 169.

5. Oswald Chambers, *My Utmost for His Highest,* ed. James Reimann (Grand Rapids, MI: Discovery House Publishers, 1995), April 7.

6. Carole Lewis with Marcus Brotherton, *First Place 4 Health: Discover a New Way to Healthy Living* (Ventura, CA: Regal, 2008), p. 26.

7. Winston Churchill, "Never Give In," *The Churchill Centre and Museum at the Churchill War Rooms, London,* October 29, 1941. http://www.winstonchurchill.org/learn/speeches/speeches-of-winston-churchill/103-never-give-in (accessed September 22, 2010).

Group Prayer Requests

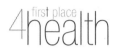

Today's Date: _____

Name	Request

Results

_____

_____

_____

_____

_____

learning from
the past

Scripture Memory Verse
*And we know that in all things God works for the good of those
who love him, who have been called according to his purpose.*
Romans 8:28

On the day of her beloved stepdaughter's wedding, Catherine Marshall, inspirational author and editor, was surprised to receive a special request from the young bride and groom. The soon-to-be newlyweds came to ask her if she would create a record of the family's spiritual history. They wanted Catherine to write down all the wisdom that she and her husband had learned on their journey so far, for the benefit of the next generation. Although, of course, the request blessed her, Catherine was more than a little overwhelmed by the magnitude of the request. How on earth could she possibly share all that God had been teaching her over a lifetime?

As she thought about it over the next few weeks, surrounded by ever-growing piles of old journals, letters and photographs, Catherine discovered something:

> I saw that the road of life I had traveled was no straight line as it
> so often appears from the wedding altar; rather it had many a
> turn and twist and bump and detour. More significantly, I real-
> ized that even Christians do not arrive at any goodness or ma-
> turity all at once. Our life is always a walk. Even on the straight
> stretches, for me there had often been such heavy fog that I had
> to go forward by faith alone that Jesus *was* with me leading the

way. And every time where I had met God had not been on the easy straightaways, but on the turns when I had least expected the revelation of His presence. . . . In searching for God's purpose—the reasons behind events—I saw that whenever I had come to Jesus stripped of pretensions, with a needy spirit, ready to listen to Him and to receive what He had for me, He had met me at my point of need. I have met God at moments where the straight road turns . . . and He has picked me up, wiped away my tears, and set me back on the path of life.[1]

Catherine's story illustrates the beauty, the blessing, of perspective—being able to look back at the lessons we've learned in the past and apply those truths to our lives today.

Day 1 LESSONS FROM THE PAST

God, open my eyes to see Your hand in my life. Show me where You have been at work behind the scenes, along the way, at every twist and turn. Amen.

In the book of Deuteronomy (*deutero* means "repetition"), Moses retells the story of everything that had happened to the Israelites—all the lessons they had learned from the time they were delivered from slavery in Egypt until they arrived at the Promised Land. Look up Deuteronomy 8:1-2. Why did God lead His people out of Egypt and into the desert?

_____

_____

_____

Of course, God already knew what was in His people's hearts, but *they* needed to know. They needed to see it. According to Deuteronomy 8:3-5, what else did they need to learn? (There are at least four things.)

1. _____

2. _____

3. _____

4. _____

Sometimes it takes a crisis, a hardship or a difficulty to get our attention—to open our eyes to something in our lives that is off balance. How has God gotten your attention lately? How did He draw you to the First Place 4 Health program?

_____

_____

_____

_____

The Israelites had all but forgotten their culture, their heritage, their faith. The former slaves were not yet strong enough to stand on their own as a nation. So God led them into the desert, to test them and teach them and train them. He promised that if they would faithfully obey His commandments, they would be His very own—His Chosen People. He would bless them and protect them and provide for them.

But the people didn't trust God; they constantly questioned Him and doubted Him. Their rebellion and disobedience turned what should have been a 12-day trip to the Promised Land into 40 years of wandering in circles under the hot desert sun. Even so, God did not abandon them. Like a loving Father, He disciplined them—and then comforted them—time and time again. Flip back a few pages to Deuteronomy 1:30-31. What beautiful word picture did Moses use to describe how God was with His people, even in their darkest days?

_____

_____

_____

_____

Moses spoke to a new generation of God's people. Their parents and grandparents had lost their chance to enter the Promised Land, but this new generation would move into it. An incredible adventure lay ahead of them. How could the new generation be sure that God would watch over them? What evidence did they have of this (see verse 31)?

_____

_____

_____

_____

What can we learn from the Israelites' story?

_____

_____

_____

_____

Father, thank You for carrying me—whether I realized it or not—through the most difficult times in my life. Help me to rest in Your arms today. Amen.

Day 2 — THE SOVEREIGNTY OF GOD

Lord, Your thoughts are higher than my thoughts, Your ways higher than my ways. Help me not to lean on my own understanding but trust in You. Amen.

This week's memory verse is one that has both comforted and challenged believers for centuries. What exactly does "God works *all things* for *good*" mean? Looking back, we've experienced some pretty unhappy things. Heart-breaking things. Evil things. There are shameful things we've done and shameful things that have been done to us. Can it be that things that make no earthly sense somehow have heavenly purpose and meaning? How is this possible?

The answer lies in the sovereignty of God. According to the dictionary, the word "sovereignty" means having supreme, unlimited power or authority, complete control. To be sovereign is to be preeminent; indisputable; greatest in degree; utmost or extreme; above all others in character, importance and excellence. Look up Colossians 1:15-20 and list what you learn about Jesus in each of the following verses:

Scripture	What you learn about Jesus
verse 15	
verse 16	
verse 17	
verse 18	
verse 19	
verse 20	

Because Jesus is all of these things, although evil is prevalent and we live in a fallen world, He has the power and the authority and the ability to cause all things to work together for our good—just as it says in Romans 8:28. Remember that when God talks about our good, He doesn't mean our immediate comfort or happiness. He means that He is making us more and more like Jesus, which will ultimately give us the greatest joy now and in eternity. But this promise is not for everyone:

> [This promise] can be claimed only by those who love God and are called according to His purpose . . . [those who receive Christ] . . . Such people have a new perspective, a new mindset on life. They trust in God, not life's treasures; they look for their security in heaven, not on earth; they learn to accept, not resent, pain and persecution because God is with them.[2]

Author, preacher and Bible teacher John Piper points out that God was able to take the most "spectacular" sin (the greatest evil, the most wicked injustice) in the history of the world—the crucifixion of Jesus—and use it to triumph over the devil, redeem His children and glorify His Son.[3] Read Colossians 2:13-15. According to verse 13, how did God demonstrate His awesome power on our behalf?

_____

_____

_____

_____

What did He do with the evidence of our guilt, the obstacle or barrier between us (see verse 14)?

_____

_____

_____

_____

How did He celebrate His victory (see verse 15)?

_____

_____

_____

_____

This metaphor suggests a victorious Roman general leading his captives—the physical evidence of his complete and total victory—through the streets for all the people to see. What question did God ask in Jeremiah 32:27? What is the answer?

_____

_____

_____

_____

Unto the King eternal, immortal, invisible, the only God, be honor and glory forever and ever. Amen.

SOVEREIGN OVER SUFFERING

Father, thank You that nothing comes my way without first passing through Your hands. Your love guides me and shields me and saves me. Amen.

We may have been through some very difficult and painful experiences in our past. We may be going through some very difficult and painful experiences right now. Read James 1:2-4. According to this passage, how should believers respond to trials and tribulations? Ultimately, what purpose does this serve?

_____

_____

_____

_____

_____

Our suffering gives us the opportunity to identify in a small way with the suffering that Jesus experienced on our behalf (see 1 Peter 4:13). It causes us to focus on the things that are truly important—things that are eternally significant. It teaches us to look to Jesus for comfort and strength, which enables us to comfort and strengthen others in Him (see 2 Corinthians 1:3-5). It also gives us authority in our witness.

Betsie ten Boom, the sister of Corrie ten Boom, anticipated the day when their experiences in Nazi concentration camps would provide them with amazing opportunities to testify to the life-changing power of the gospel:

> The most important part of our task will be to tell everyone who will listen that Jesus is the only answer to the problems that are disturbing the hearts of men and nations. We will have the right to speak because we can tell from our experience that His light is more powerful than the deepest darkness. How wonderful that the reality of His presence is greater than the reality of the hell about us.[5]

Read Hebrews 12:7-11. What is another reason for, or purpose, in our suffering (see verses 7-9)?

_____

_____

_____

Why does God discipline us (see verse 10)?

_____

_____

_____

_____

What does this discipline produce in us or for us (see verse 11)?

_____

_____

_____

What might that look like in your life today?

_____

_____

_____

_____

What was one gift, one prize, one treasure—an invaluable life lesson or particularly meaningful experience—that God has given you as a result of the pain and suffering you've been through?

_____

_____

_____

_____

God, help me not to grow discouraged in times of trouble, but to look to You and learn from You. Amen.

SOVEREIGN OVER SIN

*Lord, forgive me for my sins, for the times when I fall short of Your righteous
and holy standards. I want to do better. Help me to do better. Amen.*

We may believe that God can work in and through the hardships that
have come to us through no fault of our own. But what about the suffering we bring on ourselves—the painful consequences of our poor
choices and our un-Christlike attitudes and behaviors? The Bible assures
us that yes, in these things, too, God is sovereign. He is able to bring
good from our worst mistakes, our most disappointing failures. He
causes even our sinfulness to serve His purposes. In fact, in Romans 3:5,
the apostle Paul explained that our unrighteousness brings out God's
righteousness more clearly! According to Galatians 3:24, what was the
purpose of God's law all along?

So the very thing that condemns us—our inability to keep God's commandments—is the thing He uses to help us see our sinfulness and our
need of the Savior! Read the story of the sinful woman in Luke 7:36-50.
What did Jesus say is the moral of the story—the message for the rest of us?

How has your faith brought you peace?

An awareness of our own shortcomings, our own weaknesses, our own failings can keep us from the sin of pride and help us to have compassion for others. Read the story of the woman caught in adultery in John 8:1-11. What was Jesus' admonition to the Pharisees calling for her execution?

_____

_____

_____

_____

Why do you think "the older ones" were the first to leave (verse 9)?

_____

_____

_____

_____

While we don't want to dwell on the mistakes of our past, we do want to remember what we've learned from them; otherwise, we will make those same mistakes over and over again. What are some of the lessons you have learned from your own struggles?

_____

_____

_____

_____

How might these lessons help you on your First Place 4 Health journey?

_____

_____

_____

_____

_____

God, thank You that Your grace is greater than my sin. Even in my failures and mistakes, Your glory shines. With all my heart, I worship You! Amen.

SOVEREIGN IN LOVE

Day 5

"Search me, O God, and know my heart; test me and know my anxious thoughts. See if there is any offensive way in me, and lead me in the way everlasting" (Psalm 139:23-24). Amen.

Read Psalm 103:13-14. How do these verses describe God's heart toward each of us?

_____

_____

_____

_____

_____

Why is He tender and merciful with us?

_____

_____

_____

_____

Turn to Psalm 139. According to verses 1-4, just how well does God know us? What does He know?

_____

_____

_____

_____

How does He know these things (see verses 5-16)?

_____

_____

_____

_____

_____

Why is it good news that anything that happens to us is not a surprise to God (see verse 16)?

_____

_____

_____

How does this good news relate to your journey with First Place 4 Health?

_____

_____

_____

_____

Be encouraged: Before you were even born, God saw that you would be where you are today, and He determined that He would use this experience to accomplish something significant in your heart and life—something precious, something purposeful, something of great value for all eternity!

Lord, help me to make the most of this opportunity, to learn all I can from this experience. Use it in my life in a powerful way. In Jesus' name, amen.

Day 6 · REFLECTION AND APPLICATION

Jesus, I want Your beauty to be revealed in me. I trust You, even when I don't understand. I know You have a purpose and a plan for me. Amen.

Our memory verse, Romans 8:28, reveals that even though we might not understand why God does what He does, we *can* trust that He is working for our good. We cannot always see His purpose and plan, because our thoughts are not like God's thoughts, but one day we will learn the reasons. Here is an anonymous believer's reflection on the profound and powerful biblical truth found in Romans 8:28:

My life is but a weaving between my Lord and me.
I cannot choose the colors He works so steadily.

Oft time He weaves in sorrow and I, in foolish pride,
Forget He sees the upper and I, the underside.

Not 'til the loom is silent and the shuttles cease to fly,
Will God unroll the tapestry, and explain the reason why.
The dark threads are as needed in Heaven's skillful hand,
As the threads of gold and silver in the pattern He has planned.

Look up Romans 8:28 in your Bible and keep reading through verse 39. From this passage of Scripture, what can we learn about the heartaches and hardships we've been through in the past? (Regardless of how we felt at the time, what do we now know is true?)

How can we apply this to the challenges we face in the future?

What assurance from this passage is most meaningful to you today? Why?

How will this truth help you with the difficulties you encounter this week?

*Thank You, Father, that You can take all the heartache I've been through
and turn it into something beautiful to You. You are amazing! Amen.*

REFLECTION AND APPLICATION

Lord, help me to remember the lessons You've taught me so far, and help me to apply them to the challenges I face today. In Jesus' name, amen.

As Joshua led the Israelites into the Promised Land, God did many amazing and wondrous things to demonstrate His power and love—to show them that He was with them and would bless them in the new land. When the people arrived at the banks of the Jordan River, the river was at its fullest. But as the priests carrying the Ark of the Covenant stepped into the water at the river's edge, the flow of water miraculously ceased. It was cut off upstream, and all the people were able to walk across the riverbed as if it were dry land.

While the priests stood in the riverbed, Joshua sent the leaders of the twelve tribes back to the riverbed, commanding each of them to gather a large stone. "We will use these stones to build a memorial," he said. "In the future your children will ask, 'What do these stones mean to you?' Then you can tell them, 'They remind us that the Jordan River stopped flowing when the Ark of the Lord's Covenant went across.' These stones will stand as a permanent memorial among the people of Israel" (see Joshua 4:6-7).

A memorial is a way to remember something precious or sacred, something historic, something vitally important. People all over the world still build memorials today. It's a wonderful tradition each of us can carry on in our own hearts and with our own families.[6]

Read Psalm 71:15-18 and Psalm 77:11-14. What will the psalmist tell about? What does he promise to do?

_____

_____

_____

_____

_____

Read Psalm 77:11-14. Why does remembering the past give a person hope?

_____

_____

_____

_____

_____

_____

Do something special this week to create a lasting memory of one of these experiences. Write about the experience in a letter, journal or scrapbook, put it to music, or post it on a blog. Tell the story to your friends and family—especially your children and grandchildren. Relive the experience over and over in your heart so that you'll never forget what the Lord has done for you!

Give thanks to God for His awesome power and amazing love. Ask Him for an opportunity to share a story of His faithfulness with someone in your life today.

Lord Jesus, thank You for how far You have brought me and for all the things You have taught me. I'm in awe of Your love and Your faithfulness. Amen.

Notes

1. Catherine Marshall, *Meeting God at Every Turn: A Spiritual Autobiography* (Lincoln, VA: Chosen Books, 1980), pp. 13-14.
2. *The Life Application Study Bible* (Carol Stream, IL: Tyndale House Publishers, 2005), note on Romans 8:28, p. 1895.
3. John Piper, *Spectacular Sins: And Their Global Purpose in the Glory of Christ* (Wheaton, IL: Crossway Books, 2008), p. 33.
4. Kenneth Barker, gen. ed., *The NIV Study Bible* (Grand Rapids, MI: Zondervan Publishing House, 2002), note on Colossians 2:15, p. 1855.
5. Bestie ten Boom, quoted in Corrie ten Boom, *The Hiding Place* (Rantoul, IL: Crossings Book Club, 1984), p. 204.
6. Christin Ditchfield, *Take It to Heart: Sixty Meditations on God and His Word* (Wheaton, IL: Crossway Books, 2005), pp. 50-51.

Group Prayer Requests

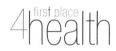

Today's Date: _____

Name	Request

Results

_____

_____

_____

_____

_____

_____

living in the present

SCRIPTURE MEMORY VERSE

He has showed you, O man, what is good. And what does the LORD require of you? To act justly and to love mercy and to walk humbly with your God.

MICAH 6:8

Looking to the future—keeping our eyes on the prize—and anticipating achieving our goals can be motivating. However, looking too far ahead can be de-motivating if it turns into pressure to reach our goals by a specific date, or into dread over all the work we have ahead of us and how far we still have to go, or into fear that we won't be able to stick with it and see it through. Our journey has barely begun, and yet some of us may already be saying, "I don't think I can do this. I'll never make it!"

For others of us, the finish line seems so far away that we're tempted to cheat—to return to our old unhealthy lifestyle—for a few days or a few weeks, thinking we can make up the lapse with shortcuts (diet pills, fasting, super-restricted calorie counts or massive amounts of exercise) later on. Of course, we're only cheating ourselves. When the future comes, we find that every wrong turn has only made getting back on track that much harder.

If we want to make real progress, we can't live in the past or the future. We've got to live in the present, facing each challenge and fighting each battle as it comes. Remember that "what leads to lasting success is making a series of small, positive choices every day."[1] We've got to focus on being obedient to God in *this* moment, asking Him for what we need to be victorious today. He promises that when we do, His answer will be "yes!" (see Matthew 7:7-8; Luke 11:9-10).

HONOR GOD

Lord, thank You for providing everything I need today—all of the wisdom, all of the grace, all of the strength, all of the peace. Amen.

An old adage states, "Yesterday is history. Tomorrow is a mystery. Today is a gift. That's why it is called the present."

Often, we feel pulled in a hundred different directions. We have to-do lists a mile long—so many commitments, obligations and responsibilities. We're not always sure that we're using our time wisely, that we've made the best choices, that our priorities are in the right place. We're not always even sure that the information we've used to make our choices is trustworthy. What if we're doing *this*, when we should be doing *that*?

We want whatever we do and whatever we choose to be pleasing to God. We want our lives to honor Him. We want to make the most of the time He has given us and to accomplish the things He wants us to accomplish. But how can we know what those things are? Look at this week's memory verse in Micah 6:8. How can we know what God wants us to accomplish?

_____

_____

_____

_____

_____

We don't have to wonder what God wants from us or how He wants us to live. He tells us in His Word! As author A. W. Tozer points out, we only need to respond to God's urging:

> God is here. The whole universe is alive with His life. And He is no strange or foreign God, but the familiar Father of our Lord Jesus Christ whose love has for these thousands of years enfolded the sinful race of men. And always He is trying to get our attention, to reveal Himself to us, to communicate with us.[2]

The Bible may not specifically address each circumstance or situation we face, but it gives plenty of guidelines and principles to help us determine what God's will is for us. And we're not left to our own devices to figure out how to apply these principles. List the three basic behaviors or attitudes God wants to see in us, according to Micah 6:8.

1. _____

2. _____

3. _____

In which of the above broad categories would you put the following more specific instructions?

_____ The Ten Commandments (see Exod. 20:3-17)

_____ The Shema—The Jewish Confession of Faith (see Deut. 6:4-9; Mark 12:30)

_____ The Golden Rule (see Matthew 22:39; Luke 10:27)

Now look up Deuteronomy 30:11-14: What does God promise about His commandments?

_____

_____

_____

Read Psalm 119:9-11. According to this passage, what is the result of "living according to [God's] word"?

_____

_____

_____

How do you avoid sinning and thus attain victory?

_____

_____

_____

How do you hide God's Word in your heart?

_____

_____

_____

_____

Look up James 1:5. If you have trouble figuring out how to apply the principles of the Bible, what should you do?

_____

_____

_____

_____

Reading and studying God's Word are paramount to your success every day, every week in your First Place 4 Health journey and in your journey as a Christian. And Scripture memorization will ensure that God's Word is available to you whenever you need it.

Father, I want my choices to reflect my commitment to You. Please give me the wisdom to act justly, love mercy and walk humbly with You. Amen.

Day 2 DON'T WAVER

Lord, teach me Your ways. Show me how to walk in obedience to Your Word today. Speak, Lord, for Your servant is listening. Amen.

Years ago, bestselling author Dr. Gary Chapman wrote a book called _The Five Love Languages,_ in which he observed that people give and receive love in different ways (words of affirmation, quality time, acts of service, receiving gifts, and physical touch). Each of us has our own primary love language—the one that we most often speak and most easily understand. Chapman says if we want someone to feel loved, we've got to learn to speak his or her language. The Bible tells us that God's love language is obedience. Jesus said, "If you love me, you will obey what I command" (John 14:15). While there are other ways we can express our love for Him, the one that means the most to Him is to do what He says!

Sometimes we're tempted to offer Him what we would like to give or what we are willing to give, rather than what He has asked for. The gift we want to offer may even appear to be a huge sacrifice. But God makes it very clear that "to obey is better than sacrifice" (1 Samuel 15:22). The context in which this week's memory verse is found reinforces this truth (see Micah 6:6-8). If we truly love God, we will show it by obeying His Word. Read John 14:21. What does Jesus promise to those who love and obey Him?

_____

_____

_____

According to Deuteronomy 10:12-13, what does God ask of us? (There are five things in this passage.)

1. _____

2. _____

3. _____

4. _____

5. _____

Why does God ask this of us (see verse 13)?

_____

_____

_____

Someone once observed that every one of God's commandments is designed either to protect us or provide for us—or both. Look up Psalm 119, often described as a passionate love poem written to God's Word. What does the psalmist tell us in the following verses about people who follow God's commands?

Scripture	What the verse says about people who follow God's commands
verses 1-2	
verse 4	
verse 14	
verse 16	
verse 24	

In yesterday's study, we read James 1:5, which encouraged us to ask God for wisdom. The next verse, James 1:6, urges us to believe in and trust God's Word, without wavering. This is important because wavering implies that we are not certain about what we should do and what we should believe:

> A mind that wavers is not completely convinced that God's way is best. It treats God's Word like any human advice, and it retains the option to disobey. It vacillates between allegiance to subjective feelings, the world's ideas, and God's commands. If your faith is new, weak, or struggling, remember that you can trust God. Then be loyal to Him.[3]

Is there an area of obedience to God in which you've been wavering lately? Confess it to God and ask His forgiveness. Pray that He will once again confirm His Word to you and help you to obey.

Father, You are always faithful and good and loving toward me.
I worship You and praise Your holy name! Amen.

ACT JUSTLY

Father, thank You for showing me what is good and what You desire from me. I want to please You in all that I say and do. In Jesus' name, amen.

What does it mean to "act justly"? At first glance, it may seem like a rather lofty concept, particularly if we think of it as delivering justice to the wicked or standing up for justice on behalf of the poor, the needy and the oppressed—in the interests of "justice being served." And perhaps on some level, that is a part of it. But at the most basic level, to act justly means to do what is right: Be true to God, be true to yourself, be true to others. Live a life of integrity. What does a life of integrity look like? For an example, turn to the Ten Commandments given in Exodus 20:3-17. In the space provided below, rewrite each "you shall not" as a positive "I shall" statement.

1. I shall _____
2. I shall _____
3. I shall _____
4. I shall _____
5. I shall _____
6. I shall _____
7. I shall _____
8. I shall _____
9. I shall _____
10. I shall _____

What are some other right things you know that God wants you to do right now? Make your answers personal and specific to you. (If you need ideas, see Romans 12:1-2,9-21.)

_____

_____

_____

_____

Why do you think God wants us to act justly or, in other words, "be holy"? What should our motivation be?

_____

_____

_____

Now we need to apply these truths to our First Place 4 Health journey. Look up 1 Corinthians 10:31 and Philippians 3:18-20. What kind of attitude should we have toward food and eating? What role should food play in our lives—and what role shouldn't it play?

_____

_____

_____

_____

Why is it important to eat right, exercise and be as healthy as we can be? Why is that a way "to act justly"?

_____

_____

_____

_____

God is calling us to respond to Him in faith, action, love and obedience. It's not about special diets, weighing and measuring food, how long you exercise each day, or checking off boxes on your Live It Tracker. These are merely tools to help you achieve the ultimate goal: a personal, loving, intimate and interactive relationship with Jesus! Anything you do—or fail to do—that hinders that relationship wages war against your soul.[4] So make a commitment today to act justly—to do what is right, what is good, and what leads to victory!

God, I want to live a life of integrity, one that reflects Your righteousness and Your holiness. Help me to always act justly and be holy. Amen.

LOVE MERCY

Thank You, Jesus, for Your mercy and grace. Your love is better than life! Amen.

One of the things God asks of us—one of the things He *requires* of us—is that we love mercy as much as He does. The dictionary defines "mercy" as "the feeling which motivates compassion; a disposition to be kind and forgiving, especially to those under one's power; something for which to be thankful, a blessing." Read Psalm 103:8-14. How does this passage describe the character and nature of God (see verse 8)?

_____

_____

_____

How does God demonstrate His mercy (see verses 10,12)?

_____

_____

_____

Why does He do this (see verses 11,13-14)?

_____

_____

_____

God understands our human frailty. He sympathizes with our weakness. Yet He calls us to a higher standard. He shows us a better way. Look up Ephesians 5:1-2. What are we to do, and why?

_____

_____

_____

In our quest for obedience—in our passion for righteousness—we must be careful not to become legalistic or pharisaical. One woman found that when she lost weight, she also lost compassion for others who struggled with obesity. Her pride in her accomplishment caused her to look down on those who to her clearly weren't trying or hadn't yet discovered the determination, self-control and self-discipline necessary to do what she had done. The Scripture warns that pride comes before a fall (see Proverbs 16:18). To the woman's great shame and embarrassment, it wasn't long before she regained all of the weight she had lost. Talk about a humbling experience! Read Luke 6:36-37. What two things did Jesus tell us to do?

1. _____
2. _____

What two things did Jesus tell us not to do?

1. _____
2. _____

What is our motivation?

_____
_____
_____

James 2:13 warns, "There will be no mercy for those who have not shown mercy to others. But if you have been merciful, God will be merciful when he judges you" (*NLT*). According to Colossians 3:13, why should we forgive those who have wronged us?

_____
_____
_____
_____

As C. S. Lewis once wrote, "To be a Christian means to forgive the inexcusable, because God has forgiven the inexcusable in you."[5] Extending forgiveness is not easy, but it's something we have to do. We can't hold others' sins against them, while asking God not to hold our sins against us. As someone once said, holding on to resentment is like drinking poison and waiting for the other person to die! Note that bitterness and unforgiveness are two powerful emotions that can drive us to overeat as we use food to stuff them or silence them. How much better to bring those things before the Lord, confess our own sin in harboring those emotions, and ask for His help to forgive the sins of others!

Lord, I know how much I need Your mercy, Your forgiveness and Your grace.
Help me to show Your mercy and forgiveness and grace to others. Amen.

WALK HUMBLY

Day 5

Thank You, God, for teaching me Your ways. You always want what's best for me—You love me too much to leave me the way I am.

What does it mean to walk humbly with our God? It means to walk reverently. Respectfully. Obediently. Remembering how great He is and how small we are. Gratefully. Look up Psalm 25:4-10. What is the psalmist's prayer? What does he ask God to do (see verses 4-5)?

_____

_____

_____

_____

What does the psalmist ask God to remember (see verse 6)?

_____

_____

_____

What does he ask Him to forget (see verse 7)?

_____

_____

_____

According to this psalm, how can we learn to walk humbly with God (see verses 4-5,9)?

_____

_____

_____

Now turn to Matthew 11:28-30. How did Jesus describe Himself (see verse 29)? What did He offer us?

_____

_____

_____

Understand that in this word picture, Jesus isn't the farmer driving the team. He's the other ox—the older, wiser, more experienced, more mature "animal," paired with the young ox (us). He is the One who knows the path, takes the lead and sets the pace. All we have to do is keep in step, stay connected and follow His lead. Why does "working" with Jesus require humility on our part?

_____

_____

_____

_____

As Carole Lewis has written, "Lasting weight loss is dependent on our relationship with God. We can struggle and sweat all we want, and we can count calories and climb stairs, but until we learn to trust Him fully with our life—until we rest in Him and let Him lead—we will never experience lasting success in this area."[6] Read 1 Peter 5:5-7. What are the benefits of submitting ourselves to God and humbling ourselves before Him?

_____

_____

_____

_____

Do you have any cares to cast on God today? If so, come humbly before Him and ask Him for His wisdom, His guidance and His help.

Lord, You are so gentle and kind and patient with me. Help me to respond to You with a heart that is eager to hear and obey. In Jesus' name, amen.

REFLECTION AND APPLICATION

Day
6

Jesus, You've done so much to show Your love for me. Help me to show my love for You today. Amen.

Think about how you might apply this week's memory verse to each aspect of your life—each goal you have set for yourself for the course of this study. How can you "act justly" as it pertains to your emotional health, spiritual health, mental health and physical health? (Note that there may be many answers, but try to focus on one thing in each area that God has been impressing on your heart.)

_____

_____

_____

How can you show that you "love mercy" in each of these areas? (It may be an attitude or a specific behavior toward yourself or others.)

_____

_____

_____

How can you "walk humbly with your God" in each of these areas?

_____

_____

_____

Father, I know that what You are asking is not too difficult for me or beyond my reach. Help me choose to obey Your Word today and every day. Amen.

REFLECTION AND APPLICATION

Lord, help me not to be discouraged by the length of the journey or the challenges I face along the way. Give me strength for this new day. Amen.

After 70 years of captivity and exile in Babylon, God's people—a remnant, a small group of survivors—were finally allowed to return to Israel to rebuild their homeland. At first it must have seemed to them like a "mission impossible." But through the prophet Zechariah, God urged His people not to "despise this day of small beginnings" (Zechariah 4:10, *THE MESSAGE*).

God told them not to look down on the first steps they had taken to rebuild His Temple, not to grow discouraged by the enormity of the task and not to feel as if their accomplishments were paltry and their efforts feeble. The work they had done might seem insignificant to them—but God was in it. He would give them the strength to finish the task. And one day, they would stand back in awe at all He had accomplished in them and through them.

God's word to the Israelites is an important reminder for us today. Sometimes our own little efforts might not seem like much to us—our attempts at rebuilding our bodies (our temple of the Holy Spirit), our attempts at obedience and ministry and service and sacrifice. They don't always seem to make much difference. And they're not nearly as impressive as we had hoped they would be. Perhaps they even pale in comparison to the achievements of others. But God sees our heart. He knows what each of those steps cost us, how hard fought each battle really was. And He can bless and multiply our efforts in ways we can't even begin to imagine. As Hudson Taylor, a famous missionary to China, once observed, "A little thing is a little thing, but faithfulness in little things is a great thing."[7]

One day, we too will stand back in awe at all that God has accomplished in us and through us! So take a few moments to list some of the things you have accomplished this week—acts of obedience, steps that you've taken toward your goals. The "little things" may be as simple, as seemingly small or insignificant as resisting a particular temptation or choosing to exercise one day when you didn't feel like it. Never mind if you gave in to other temptations this week or didn't exercise as much as you planned. A victory is a victory!

_____

_____

_____

_____

Remember that sometimes the biggest victory is that *you're still here*. You haven't quit. You're not giving up. You're still showing up, day after day. That in itself is an accomplishment! Conclude this week's session by reading the encouragement God gives us in Galatians 6:9, and write this passage in your own words in the space below.

_____

_____

_____

_____

Dear God, thank You for each and every victory, each wise choice, each posi-tive step. Help me to keep moving forward. In Jesus' name, amen.

Notes

1. Carole Lewis with Marcus Brotherton, *First Place 4 Health: Discover a New Way to Healthy Living* (Ventura, CA: Regal Books, 2008), p. 39.
2. A. W. Tozer, *The Pursuit of God* (Camp Hill, PA: Christian Publications, Inc., 1993), p. 67.
3. *The Life Application Study Bible* (Carol Stream, IL: Tyndale House Publishers, 2005), note on James 1:6, p. 2091.
4. *Simple Ideas for Healthy Living* (Ventura, CA: Gospel Light, 2008), p. 40.
5. C. S. Lewis, *The Quotable Lewis*, eds. Wayne Martindale and Jerry Root (Wheaton, IL: Tyndale Publishers, Inc., 1989), p. 221.
6. Carole Lewis, *First Place 4 Health*, p. 93.
7. Hudson Taylor, quoted in A. J. Broomhall, *Hudson Taylor and China's Open Century, Book Four: Survivors' Pact* (London: Hodder and Stroughton, 1984), p. 154.

Group Prayer Requests

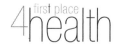

Today's Date: _____

Name	Request

Results

_____

_____

_____

_____

_____

_____

Week Five

leaning on
Jesus

Scripture Memory Verse
But he said to me, "My grace is sufficient for you, for my power is made perfect in weakness." Therefore I will boast all the more gladly about my weaknesses, so that Christ's power may rest on me.
2 Corinthians 12:9

Do you ever feel like a failure in your relationship with Christ? Is there an area of your life where it seems that victory escapes you? For many of us, it's having a healthy attitude toward food. For others, it's controlling our temper or focusing on the right priorities. All of these require us to exercise self-control and discipline. We struggle to overcome temptation and make good choices, but we seem to keep falling on our face. We've begged God to help us in these areas, but for some reason He doesn't seem to hear us. He doesn't seem to answer our prayers. He has yet to deliver us. We wonder if we're doomed to lose our battle again and again.

In 2 Corinthians 12:7-10, the apostle Paul talks about wrestling with a battle of his own, "a thorn in [his] flesh." A thorn is irritating and painful. And as long as it's stuck there, the pain is constant and so distracting that it's hard to think of anything else. It can keep a person from doing things that need to be done. Paul says of his own thorn:

Three times I pleaded with the Lord to take it away from me. But he said to me, "My grace is sufficient for you, for my power is made perfect in weakness." Therefore I will boast all the more gladly of my weaknesses, so that Christ's power may rest on me.

That is why, for Christ's sake, I delight in weaknesses, in insults, in hardships, in persecutions, in difficulties. For when I am weak, then I am strong.

Although we don't always understand the whys and wherefores, Scripture promises us that God can and will use all of our "thorns" for His glory. Our struggles humble us and keep us daily on our knees. Our very human weakness is an opportunity for God's power to work in us and through us. Don't give up. Learn to lean on Him, on His mercy and grace. For when we are weak, He is strong.

Day 1

ADMITTING OUR WEAKNESSES

Father, help me to remember today to rely on Your strength and not on my own. I can do all things through You! Amen.

In Romans 7:18-19, Paul says, "I know that nothing good lives in me, that is, in my sinful nature. For I have the desire to do what is good, but I cannot carry it out. For what I do is not the good I want to do; no, the evil I do not want to do—this I keep on doing." Can you relate?

At times we may be shocked—horrified—humbled by our own weaknesses, our own sinfulness. But God isn't shocked. He isn't even surprised. He knows very well how weak and frail we are. After all, He made us! So what was He thinking? If we're such a mess, why does He bother with us? Look up 1 Corinthians 1:26-31. What words and phrases in this passage describe the people that God has called—the people He chooses to use?

_____

_____

_____

Why does God do this (see verses 27-29)?

_____

_____

_____

Where do our righteousness, our holiness and our redemption come from—who do we boast in (see verses 30-31)?

_____

_____

_____

Read 2 Corinthians 4:6-7. What do we as believers have inside of us, and what are we supposed to do with it?

_____

_____

_____

Our flesh—our bodies—are "jars of clay," or, as author Patsy Clairmont likes to say, "cracked pots": "Picture an empty pitcher with a network of cracks down the front. Now imagine that pitcher filled with light and a lid put on the top. Where does the light shine through? The cracks. That is the same way the Lord's light shines through our lives."[1]

After Jesus rose from the dead and ascended into heaven, His disciples began preaching the gospel and carrying on His ministry of healing and deliverance, just as He had told them to do. The same religious leaders who had Jesus crucified then arrested Peter and John for preaching in His name. Look up Acts 4:13. What about Peter and John astonished the religious leaders? To what did they attribute it?

_____

_____

_____

_____

Should we be discouraged by our weaknesses? Ashamed? Distressed? Why or why not?

_____

_____

_____

_____

Lord, make my life a testimony to Your awesome power. May Your light and Your glory shine through my weaknesses today. In Jesus' name, amen.

Day 2 — RELYING ON GOD'S STRENGTH

Lord, thank You for Your love, Your mercy and Your grace. Thank You for giving me Your strength to face each challenge that comes my way. Amen.

Read Hebrews 4:14-15. Jesus is our High Priest, the only One who could enter the Holy of Holies (where the presence of God dwells) and make atonement for our sins. Why is He sympathetic to our struggles with sin?

_____

_____

_____

_____

As Carole Lewis has said, "God is full of compassion. He deals gently with us. He knows what it is like to be a human being. He sent His Son, Jesus Christ, to Earth, where Jesus was tempted in every way known to mankind without giving in to those temptations. That's what makes Him our Savior and Redeemer. It also makes Him full of compassion for all the ways we are tempted to fall."[2] Romans 2:4 says that God's kindness to us leads us to repentance. According to Luke 13:3, why is it important that we confess (admit to) our sin and repent of it?

_____

_____

_____

_____

Psalm 19:11-13 describes two categories, or kinds, of sin for which we need forgiveness. What are those categories?

1. _____

2. _____

God promises to forgive both! As we continually repent and ask God for His forgiveness, we receive it. "This is what the Sovereign LORD, the Holy One of Israel, says: 'In repentance and rest is your salvation, in quietness and trust is your strength'" (Isaiah 30:15). According to Hebrews 4:16, what else do we receive when we repent?

_____

_____

_____

_____

According to Philippians 4:19, what are we promised?

_____

_____

_____

_____

Ask God specifically for the strength you need today. Consider holding out your open hands while you pray, as if to receive that strength God wants to give to you.

Thank You, Lord, that Your grace is sufficient—that You will provide everything I need today. I receive it in Jesus' name, amen.

CALLING ON GOD

Day 3

God, I know that even when I'm tempted—especially when I'm tempted—the best thing I can do is turn to You and call on You. You always answer! Amen.

Read Matthew 26:41. Why do you think Jesus instructed His disciples to "watch"?

_____

_____

_____

_____

What did Jesus tell His disciples to pray?

_____

_____

_____

_____

Why is temptation such a problem for us?

_____

_____

_____

_____

Look up 1 Corinthians 10:13. Jesus understands our struggles with sin. He understands all our trials and temptations. He feels compassion for us. He offers us His strength to help us resist temptation. According to this verse, what else does He offer to provide for us? Why?

_____

_____

_____

_____

What are your three greatest temptations or challenges—the people, places and situations—that most easily get you into trouble, or the areas in which you're most vulnerable?

1. _____

2. _____

3. _____

It's not enough to decide we _won't_ do something; we have to decide that we _will_ do something else. In other words, we have to replace a negative behavior with a positive one. Prayerfully consider what the best strategy will be for you to avoid these temptations or challenges when they arise.

The first two are provided as an example.

Temptation or challenge	Strategy for avoiding
Overeat when I am feeling frustrated	Journal about my feelings instead
Not motivated to exercise	Phone a friend or a prayer partner

Lord, thank You for providing "a way out"—a way of escape. Open my eyes to see that "exit" whenever I'm tempted today—and help me take it! Amen.

STANDING IN GOD

Day 4

Lord, lead me not into temptation, but deliver me from evil. In Jesus' precious and holy name, amen.

Sometimes, the best way to resist temptation is to avoid it! At times, we can avoid allowing ourselves to be caught off guard in a vulnerable state and avoid those situations that may tempt us beyond what we can bear. We can run fast in the opposite direction! But other times, we have to face temptation head on. In such cases, there's nothing to do but take a stand—and fight back! Read Ephesians 6:10-17. According to this passage, what kind of battle are we in? Who or what is the enemy?

_____

_____

_____

_____

What protection do we have? What does this include (see verses 13-17)?

_____

_____

_____

Most of the elements of the armor of God are *defensive* weapons—things that prepare us or protect us. Which one is an *offensive* weapon? How can we use this to fight back (see verse 17)?

_____

_____

_____

_____

In Matthew 4:1-11, Jesus modeled for us how we should handle confrontation with the enemy of our souls. Three times Satan came to Him, challenged Him and tested Him, tempting Him to sin. Perhaps Jesus could have vanquished the devil supernaturally. He was, after all, God in the flesh. But Jesus didn't use His divine power to defeat the devil—perhaps because you and I are not God, and we don't have that kind of power. Instead, Jesus used a weapon that is available to every believer, from the newest "baby" Christian to the most seasoned saint. Every time the devil tempted Him, Jesus answered, "It is written . . ." He quoted Scripture. How does Hebrews 4:12 describe this weapon?

_____

_____

_____

_____

According to 2 Corinthians 10:4-5, what does this weapon have the power to do?

_____

_____

_____

This is why Scripture memory is such an important part of your First Place 4 Health journey! How can taking every thought captive help us when we're tempted to overeat or skip a workout or disregard what God has spoken to us in some other aspect of our lives?

_____

_____

_____

_____

Father, thank You for providing Your armor to protect me and Your sword to defend me. Help me to take back some of the ground the enemy has gained in my life, and help me to stand on the truth of Your Word. Amen.

RESTING IN GOD   Day 5

Lord, thank You that I can stand in You. And when I feel as if I can't stand, thank You for letting me lean on You and rest in You. Amen.

Every one of us has moments when we are battle weary—when we feel as if we don't have the strength to stand, let alone fight. In these moments, we can draw comfort from Scriptures like Deuteronomy 33:27: "The eternal God is your refuge, and underneath are the everlasting arms." When we run to Him, He hides us safe in His arms. He carries us through the storms of life—the fiery trials—and the long, dark nights of the soul. Read Isaiah 40:28-31. According to these verses, just who is the Lord?

_____

_____

_____

Why are we safe in His arms (see verse 28)?

_____

_____

_____

_____

What does He give to the weary? To the weak (see verse 29)?

_____

_____

_____

_____

What happens to those who put their hope in Him (see verse 31)?

_____

_____

_____

_____

Hebrews 11 is sometimes called the Hall of Faith chapter of the Bible, because it tells of many of the great men and women of God whose lives were a testimony to God's amazing power and grace. None of them were perfect. They all made mistakes. But their faith and courage are an inspiration to us today. If you have time, go ahead and read through the whole chapter! Otherwise, turn to Hebrews 11:32-40. According to Hebrews 11:34, how did God help some of the faithful men and women?

_____

_____

_____

_____

Note that not everyone in the Hall of Faith experienced divine intervention or miraculous deliverance or supernatural victory. Some experienced quite the opposite! But they all persevered. They all pressed on. And together with us, they have received God's promise of salvation—His precious gift of eternal life through Jesus, His Son. And that's what matters more than anything else.

Lord, my eyes are fixed on You. You are the source of my hope,
my strength, my joy, my peace. I rest in You. Amen.

REFLECTION AND APPLICATION

Jesus, You are my strength and my shield; my heart trusts in You and I am helped. I rejoice in Your unfailing love. Amen.

Many of us have sung the old hymn "Leaning on the Everlasting Arms," which states, "What a fellowship, what a joy divine, leaning on the everlasting arms; what a blessedness, what a peace is mine, leaning on the everlasting arms."[3] It is an incredible privilege to walk with Jesus. Each day, our precious Lord and Savior invites us to learn from Him and lean on Him—to draw our strength from Him as we grow in His grace. Here are some simple, practical ways we can lean on Jesus today and every day:

- Spend time in His Word. Set aside a regular time for Bible study and prayer.
- Talk to Him throughout the day. Express your love for Him; share your hopes and dreams, your worries, your fears, your needs and the needs of others as they arise.
- Plan a personal retreat. Take some time when you can set everything else aside and focus on your relationship with Him.
- Memorize Scripture. Learn the First Place 4 Health memory verses and others that are meaningful to you. Quote them when they speak to the temptations and challenges you face.
- Post Scripture verses and other inspirational thoughts where you'll see them often.
- Be inspired wherever you are and no matter what you're doing. Fill your heart, your home, your office and your car with praise and worship music that turns your thoughts toward Him. You can also listen to the Scriptures or good, Bible-based sermons while you walk on a treadmill or while you drive to work or do errands.
- Share His love with others. Reach out and encourage someone else with a note or a phone call, or extend an invitation to get together over coffee.

- Keep going to church, your First Place 4 Health Bible study, and any other places you find fellowship, encouragement and the opportunity to grow in your faith.
- Seek godly counsel when you need it. Talk to a trusted friend or family member, a pastor or a Christian counselor—people God has placed in your life to help you!
- Go to a concert or a museum, read a good book, take a walk on the beach or gaze at the mountains. Rejoice in the beauty and creativity and splendor of the God who created or inspired the things that inspire you!
- Count your blessings—and give thanks!
- Make a list of the reasons you began this journey and the things you hope to accomplish. Purpose in your heart to do your part, and trust God to do His.

What other ways can you think of to lean on Jesus?

_____

_____

_____

_____

Lord, give me wisdom and courage to face each trial or temptation that comes my way today. The victory is mine, but the battle belongs to You. Amen.

Day 7 — REFLECTION AND APPLICATION

Lord, my hope is in You, my faith is in You, my trust is in You. May my life bring You glory and honor today. In Jesus' name, amen.

When things go well, we're often quick to take credit. We think we've achieved the victory on our own—with our own talent and skill, our own intelligence, our own effort, our own willpower and our own strength. But the truth is that without God, we can do nothing. We're completely helpless and doomed to fail!

Sometimes God allows us to face the most challenging trials when we feel weakest, when our resources are exhausted and when our friends and allies are nowhere in sight, so we'll realize just how helpless we are and how desperately we need Him. When He comes to our rescue, we see how strong, powerful and mighty He is—how good and faithful and loving and kind. The truth of our memory verse is made evident. We see Him do things in us and through us that we could never have even dreamed.

As Joni Eareckson Tada states, "Sometime beyond all time, we'll stand together before His throne and acknowledge that He did it all . . . through His strength, in keeping with His character, by His incredible grace, and to the praise of His glory. And to think He included you and me!"[4] Of course, we don't have to wait until we're in heaven to give Him the glory for the things He has done. We can do it right here, right now.

Write a few words of prayer—a personal expression of gratitude, of praise and of worship—from your heart to His.

_____

_____

_____

_____

_____

Lord, let me be a witness for You—a testimony to the miraculous, life-changing power of Your Holy Spirit! May my boast be always in You! Amen.

Notes

1. Patsy Clairmont, *God Uses Cracked Pots* (Carol Stream, IL: Tyndale House, 1999), p. 1.
2. Carole Lewis, with Marcus Brotherton, *First Place 4 Health: Discover a New Way to Healthy Living* (Ventura, CA: Regal Books, 2008), p. 46.
3. Elisha A. Hoffman, "Leaning on the Everlasting Arms," *Timeless Truths Free Online Library,* 2002-2010. http://library.timelesstruths.org/music/Leaning_on_the_Ever lasting_Arms (accessed October 2, 2010).
4. Joni Eareckson Tada, *Secret Strength: For Those Who Search* (Portland, OR: Multnomah, 1988), p. 22.

Group Prayer Requests

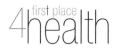

Today's Date: _____

Name	Request

Results

_____

_____

_____

_____

_____

_____

looking ahead

SCRIPTURE MEMORY VERSE

*Being confident of this, that he who began a good work in you
will carry it on to completion until the day of Christ Jesus.*

PHILIPPIANS 1:6

It is important to live in the present. We don't want to be stuck in the past or so pre-occupied with the future that we miss out on what is happening in the here and now. But there's also a danger in being short-sighted—in focusing so much on our present circumstances that we lose perspective and forget the big picture. We could begin living for this earthly life—which is temporary and fleeting at best—instead of keeping our eyes fixed on eternity.

When we lose sight of our ultimate goal, our priorities get mixed up in a hurry. We store up our treasure here on earth, instead of in heaven. We sacrifice eternal blessings and rewards for immediate and temporary comforts. We focus on what we look like (or want to look like) instead of on who we are and who we are becoming. We try to earn the approval of others and forget that it's God's approval that counts.

Moses was one man who didn't have this problem. He had the right perspective, and it helped him make a critical, life-changing choice. The book of Hebrews tells us that Moses could have remained in the lap of luxury, living as a prince in Egypt and denying his heritage and the call of God on his life. It certainly would have been a lot more comfortable and convenient for him. But as Hebrews 11:24-26 says:

By faith Moses when he had grown up, refused to be known as the son of Pharaoh's daughter. He chose to be mistreated along with the people of God *rather than to enjoy the pleasures of sin for a short time*. He regarded disgrace for the sake of Christ as of greater value than the treasures of Egypt, *because he was looking ahead to his reward* (emphasis added).

On this journey to a balanced, healthy, God-honoring lifestyle, we all need that kind of vision. We need to remember what God has called us to and what He promises to those who love Him. It's why we're doing this. It's why *He's* doing this in us and through us. And He will finish what He started.

Day 1 — GOD'S PURPOSE

Lord, help me to live in the light of eternity today. May Your priorities be my priorities; Your passion, my passion; Your purpose, my calling. Amen.

Look up Romans 8:28-30. What is "the good" that God has begun in us?

_____

_____

_____

According to 1 Peter 2:20-21, how can we be like Jesus?

_____

_____

_____

Turn to 1 Peter 1:13-16. On what do we set our hope (see verse 13)?

_____

_____

_____

_____

The Bible tells us that the day is coming when Jesus will return in power and glory to judge the nations of the earth. He will accomplish everything He has purposed to do—everything ordained since the foundation of time. His work will be completed in the world and in us. Until then, what are we to do (see verses 13-15)?

_____

_____

_____

How does your participation in the First Place 4 Health program help you follow these instructions?

_____

_____

_____

What role does living a healthy, balanced lifestyle play?

_____

_____

_____

As Oswald Chambers once wrote, we should "thank God for the glorious and majestic truth that His Spirit can work the very nature of Jesus into us, if we will only obey Him!"[1]

God, please help me to have the mind of Christ. Work in my heart and life to make me more like Your precious Son. In His name, I pray. Amen.

GOD'S POWER

Day 2

Father, thank You that You are the One who will accomplish Your purposes in my life. Nothing is impossible for You! Amen.

There are times when we don't feel very Christlike—times when, frankly, we can't even imagine that we will ever be anything like Him. He is so perfect, and we are so . . . not. But God says our becoming like Christ is not only a possibility but also a promise. Every day, in every situation and circumstance, He is working in our lives to help us become more like His precious Son. He gives us opportunity after opportunity to learn and grow. And He has the power—the ability—to make it so. Look up Matthew 19:26. What does Jesus say about this power?

_____

_____

_____

_____

According to 2 Corinthians 9:8, what is God able to do for you? Why will He do this?

_____

_____

_____

_____

Now turn to 2 Peter 1:3-4. What has God given us?

_____

_____

_____

_____

Why has He given us these things (see verse 4)?

_____

_____

_____

_____

Author and missionary Lettie B. Cowman once stated, "It is the everlasting faithfulness of God that makes a Bible promise 'very great and precious.' Human promises are often worthless, and many broken promises have left broken hearts. But since the creation of the world, God has never broken a single promise to one of His trusting children."[2] Do you believe this? Do you believe the promises of God? According to Luke 1:45, what happens to those who believe God's promises?

Close your Bible study time today by praying this benediction from Ephesians 3:20-21.

Now to him who is able to do immeasurably more than all we ask or imagine, according to His power that is at work within us, to him be glory in the church and in Christ Jesus throughout all generations, forever and ever! Amen.

OUR PATIENCE

Day 3

Father, help me to trust You with the timing—the length and the duration— and the direction of my journey. Where You lead, I will follow. Amen.

Sometimes we get impatient with the process. Why is it taking so long? We don't feel like we're making any progress or enough progress. At times it may even seem as if we're going backward or around and around in circles. But God knows what He's doing. He knows the best route and the best pace for each one of us. Our journey may not look like anyone else's. But we can be sure that it's the best way for us to take. God is at work, doing so much more than we can understand or imagine. Look up Isaiah 55:8-9. What important reminder do you find here?

Now read 2 Peter 3:8-9. Why does it sometimes seem as if God is slow in keeping His promises?

_____

_____

_____

What analogy found in James 5:7-8 explains this?

_____

_____

_____

_____

In John 15:5, how did Jesus describe us in relationship to Himself?

_____

_____

_____

J. Hudson Taylor noted, "The branch of the vine does not worry, and toil, and rush here to seek for sunshine, and there to find rain. No; it rests in union and communion with the vine; and at the right time, in the right way, is the right fruit found on it. Let us so abide in the Lord Jesus." What fruit is God laboring to produce in your life right now?

_____

_____

_____

_____

Don't try to rush the process! Keep your eyes on the ultimate goal. And be patient. Let God do what He wants to do in your heart and life today.

Lord, thank You that You never give up on me. You always keep working in my life to produce the fruit that is pleasing to You. I love You! Amen.

OUR PERSEVERANCE

Lord, please be with me today. Help me to press on and persevere, no matter what challenges come my way. Keep my eyes on the prize! Amen.

The apostle Paul often compared the Christian life to running in a race: "Forgetting what is behind and straining toward what is ahead, I press on toward the goal to win the prize for which God has called me heavenward in Christ Jesus" (Philippians 3:13-14). Look up 1 Corinthians 9:24-27. How focused on "the prize"—on the finish line—does Paul say we should be? Rewrite his exhortation and encouragement in your own words.

_____

_____

_____

_____

In New Testament times, Olympic athletes received a crown of laurel leaves—a crown that would eventually wither and fade away. According to Paul, what do we receive (see verse 25)?

_____

_____

_____

Turn to James 1:2-4. Why should we rejoice when we face trials?

_____

_____

_____

_____

Why is perseverance so important (see verse 4; see also James 1:12)?

_____

_____

_____

_____

In these passages, the word "crown" is used as a symbol of our spiritual birthright—all the blessings and rewards that we inherit as children of the King, not only in this life, but also—and most especially—in the life to come. Read 2 Corinthians 4:16-18. Why shouldn't we allow ourselves to grow weary or discouraged as we run the race of faith?

_____

_____

_____

_____

On what should we focus (see verse 18)?

_____

_____

_____

_____

Oswald Chambers wrote that "perseverance is more than endurance. It is endurance combined with assurance and certainty that what we are looking for is going to happen."[3] Read Hebrews 10:23-24. What word reminds you (again) of running in a race (see verse 23)? In what specific ways can you "spur"—inspire and encourage—other runners?

_____

_____

_____

_____

Now follow some of your own suggestions! Pray and ask God to put someone on your heart that you can encourage today. Encourage that person to press on and persevere—as you persevere, too!

Father God, please help me to live in the light of eternity and share Your light with someone else today. In Jesus' name, amen.

OUR PEACE

*Lord, I don't want to be anxious about anything today. My hope and my
trust are in You. Please fill me with Your peace. In Jesus' name, amen.*

Look up Isaiah 26:3. As we believe God to complete the work that He
has begun in us, as we wait to see the fruit of His work in our hearts and
lives, and as we persevere through trials and tribulations, what does God
promise to give us?

_____

_____

_____

_____

To whom is that gift specifically given?

_____

_____

_____

_____

Read John 14:27. Where does peace come from?

_____

_____

_____

"Peace be with you" was a common Hebrew greeting, but Jesus used it in
a different way. He used "peace" to refer to the salvation He came to
bring and the total wellbeing and inner rest of the spirit in fellowship
with God. "All true peace is His gift, which the repetition emphasizes. 'I
do not give . . . as the world gives.' In its greetings of peace, the world can
only express a longing or a wish. But Jesus' peace is real and present."[4]

Furthermore, "Unlike worldly peace, which is usually defined as the
absence of conflict, this peace is confident assurance in any circumstance; with Christ's peace, we have no need to fear the present or the

future. Sin, fear, uncertainty, doubt, and numerous other forces are at war within us. The peace of God moves into our hearts and lives to restrain these hostile forces and offer comfort in place of conflict."[5] Read Philippians 4:7. How does the apostle Paul describe this peace?

_____

_____

_____

What special purpose does it serve?

_____

_____

_____

Conclude today's study by praying the benediction found in Hebrews 13:20-21. You can read it from the *New International Version* or the following version from the *Amplified Bible*. You might want to underline any particular phrases or expressions that speak to you as you pray.

> *Now may the God of peace [Who is the Author and the Giver of peace], Who brought again from among the dead our Lord Jesus, that great Shepherd of the sheep, by the blood [that sealed, ratified] the everlasting agreement (covenant, testament), strengthen (complete, perfect) and make you what you ought to be and equip you with everything good that you may carry out His will; [while He Himself] works in you and accomplishes that which is pleasing in His sight, through Jesus Christ (the Messiah); to Whom be the glory forever and ever (to the ages of the ages). Amen (so be it).*

Day
6

REFLECTION AND APPLICATION

Lord Jesus, You have not led me this far only to leave me now. I know You will continue to walk with me on this journey—every step of the way. Amen.

When you began your First Place 4 Health journey, you set some goals for each of the four areas of your life: emotional (E), spiritual (S), mental (M) and physical (P). We're now halfway through this 12-week study, so take some time to check your progress. Review the goals you recorded in Week Two. Which of these statements best reflects where you are in your journey in regard to each of your goals?

Statement	E	S	M	P
I'm right on track, and I'm going to make it!				
I can do it, but I'll have to work harder.				
I've met my goal, and I need a new one!				
I need to adjust my goal to something more doable for me right now.				

Now, in the space provided, rerecord the goals you still need to obtain and recommit yourself to accomplishing them. If you need to adjust your goals or set some new ones, use this space to do it. (For ideas or suggestions, talk to your First Place 4 Health Group Leader.)

_____

_____

_____

_____

What do you need to do (or do differently) to win the race to reach each of your goals?

_____

_____

_____

_____

Thank You, God, that You always finish what You start. You will complete the work You have begun in me for Your glory and my good. Amen.

REFLECTION AND APPLICATION

Lord, I long for the day when I will see You face to face. Your work in me
will finally be complete and we will celebrate together for all eternity!

Some people say that this life is as good as it gets. Do you believe that?

Author Randy Alcorn says it's true—if you are an unbeliever.[6] Just
think about it. For those who do not put their faith and trust in Jesus—for those who refuse His gift of salvation—this world is as close to
heaven as they will ever get. This world full of war, poverty, famine,
disease, hardship, heartache, betrayal and disappointment is as much
paradise as they will ever experience. It will only go downhill from
here . . . all the way down into hell—eternal separation from God. Far
away and far apart from anything that is good or true or kind or loving, anything pleasant or happy or beautiful, anything creative or in-
spiring and uplifting.

The good news is that for those who do choose Jesus, those who
do believe in Him and trust Him and love Him and serve Him, this
world is as close to hell as we will ever get. This is the most hardship, the
most difficulty, the most pain, the most evil we will ever face. And it's
over before we know it, gone in a flash. (Think how quickly the last year
flew by!) From here, it only gets better. We will find ourselves in a true
paradise of perfection, full of love, joy, peace, beauty, kindness and light.
We'll have all kinds of things to do, places to go, people to see—and all
will be exciting, rewarding, invigorating and fulfilling. We have so much
to look forward to!

Most importantly, we'll see Jesus face to face. We'll experience His
presence like never before. We'll bask in His light and His love. We'll be
completely set free from our sin nature. God's work in us will be complete! No more battles with temptation, no more failures, no more frustration. The victory will be ours forever!

Do you think you can make it until then? Can you get through
whatever time you've got left—not only by making the most of this life,
but also by hanging on to the hope of heaven?

Is there anything that is holding you back from believing that God is indeed doing "good work" in you? If so, what is holding you back?

_____

_____

_____

_____

In what specific ways (even if they're small) have you seen or felt God change you so that you are beginning to reflect Jesus?

_____

_____

_____

_____

Talk to God about any concerns you have. Don't get mired in the muck and mud of this earthly life. Look up and, like Jesus, look ahead to the reward. Look ahead to the joy that will be ours for all eternity.

Lord, let me be a witness for You—a testimony to the life-changing power of Your Holy Spirit. Help me to be confident that You have begun a good work in me and that You will finish what You started. Amen.

Notes

1. Oswald Chambers, *My Utmost for His Highest*, ed. James Reimann (Grand Rapids, MI: Discovery House Publishers, 1995), April 8.
2. Lettie B. Cowman, *Streams in the Desert*, ed. James Reimann (Grand Rapids, MI: Zondervan, 2008), March 8.
3. Chambers, *My Utmost for His Highest*, February 22.
4. Kenneth Barker, gen. ed., *The NIV Study Bible* (Grand Rapids, MI: Zondervan, 2002), note on John 14:27, p. 1659.
5. *The Life Application Study Bible* (Carol Stream, IL: Tyndale House Publishers, 2005), note on John 14:27, p. 1774.
6. Randy Alcorn, *Heaven* (Carol Stream, IL: Tyndale House Publishers, 2004).

Group Prayer Requests

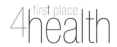

Today's Date: _____

Name	Request

Results

_____

_____

_____

_____

_____

_____

giving our
best

SCRIPTURE MEMORY VERSE
*Whatever you do, work at it with all your heart,
as working for the Lord, not for men.*
COLOSSIANS 3:23

In Matthew 21:28-31, Jesus told a story about a man who had two sons. The man went to his first son and said, "Son, go and work today in the vineyard." But the first son refused. "No, I will not," he answered. But later he changed his mind and went. Then the father went to the other son and said the same thing: "Son, go and work today in the vineyard." The other son answered, "Yes, sir, I will, sir." But he never went.

Jesus asked the crowd gathered around Him, "Which of the two sons did what his father wanted?" They answered, "The first." Jesus used this story to point out to the Pharisees—the pompous, pious religious leaders of the day—that God wants more from us than lip service. We may say all the right things. And we may say them at the right time and in the right way. But do we really mean what we say?

For example, do we really love our heavenly Father and want to do His will? Sometimes our lips say yes, but our lives say no. We are a walking contradiction, and our words are meaningless. Those around us can see the duplicity, the hypocrisy. If we want to bring glory and honor to God, it's not enough to talk the talk—we've got to walk the walk!

But there's another moral to the story we can't afford to miss. Remember that first son? The one who, in essence, threw a tantrum and initially refused to do what his father asked him to? It turns out that when all was said and done (literally!), he was the hero of the story. He was the obedient son! He had the courage to admit that he had been wrong, that his attitude—his heart—hadn't been right. And he didn't just feel badly about it. He didn't slink off into a corner to hide. He didn't wallow in his guilt. He got up and went out to the vineyard and started working. He gave it his best. In the end, he did do the job his father had asked him to do.

What a wonderful reminder that it's not too late for any of us to be the loving, obedient children that, deep down, we long to be.[1]

Day 1

WHATEVER WE DO

Lord, help me be faithful and obedient to do all that You ask of me today. In Jesus' name and for His glory, amen.

Look up Colossians 3. In many Bibles, there is a heading that summarizes the theme of each chapter. In the *New International Version*, for example, the theme of this chapter is "Rules for Holy Living." Colossians 3:5-11 tells us what *not to do*. Colossians 3:12-24 tells us what *to do*. Read Colossians 3:17, and rewrite it in your own words.

_____

_____

_____

_____

Now read this week's memory verse along with the two verses that follow it (Colossians 3:23-25). According to these verses, what should we do in the name of Jesus and for His glory (see verse 23)?

_____

_____

_____

_____

_____

Give some specific examples from your own life—things you do on a daily basis—that would fall into this category.

_____

_____

_____

_____

How are you supposed to do these things (see verses 23-24)? Why?

_____

_____

_____

While we do these things, what else are we supposed to be doing (see verse 17)?

_____

_____

_____

A lot of us do many things that we feel are "thankless jobs." Ultimately where will our "thanks"—our reward—come from (see verse 24)?

_____

_____

_____

_____

For what do we have to give thanks?

_____

_____

_____

_____

God, whatever I do, in everything I do, I want to be pleasing to You and I want to thank You. Be glorified in my life today. Amen.

ALL OUR HEART

Lord, help me not to obey You reluctantly or begrudgingly or distractedly or half-heartedly. I want to give my best for You! Amen.

Look up each of the following Scriptures and list what each one says we are to do "with all [our] heart." Then go back and draw a box around each verb, or action word.

Deuteronomy 6:5 _____

Deuteronomy 26:16 _____

Psalm 9:1 _____

Proverbs 3:5 _____

Jeremiah 29:13 _____

Ephesians 6:7 _____

Colossians 3:23 _____

How does Psalm 78:8 describe the Israelites after they left Egypt?

_____

_____

_____

_____

Read Psalm 86:11-12. What did the psalmist ask God to give him? Why is this important? What would it enable him to do?

_____

_____

_____

_____

Throughout Scripture, God calls His people to love and obey Him "wholeheartedly" or "with all your heart" (see Numbers 14:24; Deuteronomy 6:5). He even says that He is "jealous" for our love and affection (see Exodus 20:5). He wants our complete devotion. Why do you think that is?

_____

_____

_____

None of us wants to be loved—or obeyed, for that matter—half-heartedly or reluctantly or begrudgingly. This truth is the same for us as it is for God (see Revelation 3:15-16). What does Philippians 2:14-15 tell us?

_____

_____

_____

What does joyful obedience have to do with our witness for Christ (see verse 15)?

_____

_____

_____

How would you describe your obedience to God right now? Is it whole-hearted? Is it joyful? All of the time? Some of the time? Ever?

_____

_____

_____

Have you fallen into the habit of complaining about *having* to obey God in this area or that area of your life? Do you grumble and complain about *having* to eat right or *having* to exercise? *Having* to be patient or control your temper? *Having* to forgive? *Having* to resist a temptation to buy something or deny yourself something that your flesh dearly wants? If so, it's time for an attitude adjustment! Realize that these things are not things you *have* to do. These are things you *get* to do to show God that you love Him. These are things you *choose* to do to take care of your spiritual, emotional, mental and physical health—not only for your own benefit, but also for God's glory.

This week, whenever you hear yourself groan or moan and start a sentence with "Ugh, I *have* to . . ." replace it with one that expresses your desire to obey God wholeheartedly in this area of your life. You might prepare a few of these affirmations in advance. For example, "Thank You, Lord, that I can choose to forgive my sister for hurting me and that I can bring glory to You through my obedience." Or "Thank You, Lord, that You are teaching me self-discipline and self-control and that I can make healthy eating choices today."

Jesus, please give me an undivided heart, that I may walk in Your truth and joyfully, faithfully obey Your Word! Amen.

Day 3 SLAVES FOR HIM

Father, thank You that each new day is a new opportunity for me to love You and serve You with all my heart. Help me to make the most of it! In Jesus' name, amen.

Read Ephesians 6:5-9 and Colossians 3:22–4:1. After speaking to believers about how families should function, the apostle Paul addressed the relationships between slaves and their masters. Slavery was a common practice in nearly every culture during ancient times. Some slaves were prisoners of war, while others sold themselves or their family members into slavery for a period of time in order to pay off their debts. To apply the principles in these Scripture passages today, we might substitute the words "employee" and "employer" for "slave" and "master." Let's look at another way the Bible uses the imagery of slavery. Turn to Romans 6:6-7.

Why did Jesus die for us and crucify "our old self" (our old sinful nature) with Him?

_____

_____

_____

_____

Now turn to Romans 6:12-13. What does a slave to sin do?

_____

_____

_____

What are some things that want to "master" you, or control you (areas in which you struggle with temptation and/or disobedience)?

_____

_____

_____

According to verses 16-18, how do you become a slave in a spiritual sense?

_____

_____

_____

Thomas à Kempis once said, "True peace of heart . . . is found by resisting our passions, not by obeying them."[2] What sort of slave should you strive to be, and how does this happen?

_____

_____

_____

The apostle Paul frequently described himself as a "slave" to Christ, though modern translations sometimes substitute the word "servant." Whether we are servants or slaves to Christ, the point is that we no longer do as we will, but as He wills. The question is not what we want but what He wants. He is the One we ultimately answer to, and He is the One who will reward us for our obedience to Him.

Lord, it is a privilege to be Your servant, to walk in obedience to Your Word. Help me give myself fully and completely to You. Amen.

Day 4 — SACRIFICIAL OBEDIENCE

Lord Jesus, thank You for all that You sacrificed on my behalf—all that it cost You to set me free from slavery to sin. Help me to live a life worthy of Your calling. Amen.

Author and Bible teacher Lysa TerKeurst shared the following about a season in her life when God challenged her to become "radically obedient"—to learn to say yes to Him, whatever the cost, whatever the request:

Obedience becomes radical when we say, "Yes, God, whatever You want," and we mean it. We release our grip on all that we love and offer it back to Him, who loves us more. And it is into these upturned hands that God will pour out His blessings—His abundant, unexpected, radical blessings.[3]

Take a few moments and prayerfully consider whether there is something keeping you from obeying God wholeheartedly in your life today. Is there anything you need to release to Him?

_____

_____

_____

_____

What might you need to be willing to do to "open your hands"—to allow God to remove this hindrance or obstacle to obedience in your life?

_____

_____

_____

_____

Sometimes obedience requires sacrifice. If we are going to give God our best, we may have to give up other things that get in the way—even things that might otherwise be considered good. It's been said that "good things become bad things when they keep us from the best!" Turn to 1 Chronicles 21:24. King David wanted to purchase a piece of land to build an altar and offer sacrifices before the Lord. The man who owned the land volunteered to give it to him, but David refused to accept the property without paying for it. Why?

_____

_____

_____

_____

A true sacrifice costs us something. And that's what makes it meaningful. Read Luke 7:36-50. How did the sinful woman lavish her love on Jesus?

_____

_____

_____

What did it cost her?

_____

_____

_____

What motivated her to make this sacrifice? What did she receive in return (see verses 47,50)?

_____

_____

_____

What has it cost you (or would it cost you) to be obedient to God in all you do, especially in making healthy lifestyle choices?

_____

_____

_____

What have you received (or will you receive) in return?

_____

_____

_____

As Augustine once said, "God gives where He finds empty hands." So keep your eyes open, and remember that some of the blessings and rewards of obedience in one area of your life may come in another area. Often as you obey God in one thing, He blesses you in another!

Lord Jesus, show me where I need to continue to surrender myself to You. Help me to be radically obedient to You. In Your precious name, amen.

Day 5 — BLESSINGS AND REWARDS

Heavenly Father, You are so good to me—so merciful, so gracious, so kind. Thank You for pouring out Your blessings upon me. Amen.

Last week we looked ahead to the reward God has promised to those who press on and persevere and cross the finish line in the race of faith.

Let's look now at the specific rewards that are related to our obedience. Read Deuteronomy 28:1-14. What are some of the blessings listed that God promises His people?

_____

_____

_____

_____

_____

What is the often-repeated condition for these blessings (see verses 1-2, 9,13-14)?

_____

_____

_____

According to 2 Chronicles 16:9, what does God do for those whose hearts are fully committed to Him?

_____

_____

_____

_____

_____

Turn to Isaiah 55:1-2. Too often we waste our time and effort, our energy and our resources, on things that can't give us what we're looking for. They just don't satisfy us. What does God promise to those who hunger and thirst for righteousness (see also Matthew 5:6)?

_____

_____

_____

_____

Read Hosea 10:12. What happens if we sow righteousness? What will we reap?

_____

_____

_____

_____

_____

According to Philippians 4:9, what will we experience as a result of our obedience?

_____

_____

_____

_____

Now look up 2 Timothy 2:20-21. If we choose to walk in obedience to God, what will we become?

_____

_____

_____

_____

When we walk in obedience—even when it includes suffering and sacrifice—whose example are we following (see 1 Corinthians 11:1)?

_____

_____

_____

_____

_____

God, help me to choose obedience today. I believe every one of Your promises. You are always true to Your Word. Amen.

REFLECTION AND APPLICATION

Lord, thank You for the time, the energy, the gifts and talents, and all the other resources You have given me. Help me to use them for Your glory.

Another story Jesus told was about a man who was called away on business and left his servants in charge (see Matthew 25:14-30). When he gave them their assignments, he took into account their individual temperament and personality, their experience, wisdom and maturity. "To one he gave five talents of money, to another two talents, and to another one talent."

When the owner returned, he was eager to hear what his servants had done with the resources he had left in their care. The first one said, "Master, you entrusted me with five talents. See, I have gained five more." The master said to him, "Well done, good and faithful servant!"

The second servant said, "Master, you entrusted me with two talents; see, I have gained two more." Again, the master was pleased. "Well done, good and faithful servant!" Then the last servant came forward rather sheepishly. He had hidden the money, burying it in the ground. He knew his lack of initiative, his laziness, his irresponsibility was about to be exposed. Instead of admitting his mistake, though, he made excuses. He tried to shift the blame—onto his master, of all people! He called his master "hard and unforgiving," and he said that he had been afraid of what would happen if he failed. His master saw right through his excuses. He took the talent away from the unfaithful servant and sent him away in shame and disgrace.

Today, because of this story, we refer to a "talent" as a gift that someone has been given to use for their own benefit and the benefit of others. There are many different gifts, or talents, that God has given each one of us—gifts of time, energy and other resources. Some of us are more "gifted" than others in certain areas. But whether the measure of our talent is great or small, whether our opportunities to use this talent are many or (comparatively) few, what God asks is that we make the most of our talent—that we do our best with what He has given us.[4]

Think about what talent(s) God has given you. How can you be obedient and use your talent(s) to work for the Lord?

_____

_____

_____

_____

Lord, I thank You for the privilege of giving back to You—of using what You've given me to bless others and bring glory to You. Amen.

Day
7

REFLECTION AND APPLICATION

Lord, search my heart. Help me to see what You see and respond earnestly and sincerely to what You show me. In Jesus' name, amen.

In a contemplative moment, humorist Erma Bombeck once said, "When I stand before God at the end of my life, I would hope that I would not have a single bit of talent left, and could say, 'I used everything You gave me.'"[5] Take some time to think about whether you have been putting everything you have into your First Place 4 Health journey so far. Are you giving God your very best? Have you been working with all of your heart, as our memory verse says to do? Why or why not?

_____

_____

_____

_____

What about in other areas or aspects of your life? Are you walking in obedience to God? Are you using your time, your talents, your energy and efforts to accomplish His purposes for you? Why or why not?

_____

_____

_____

_____

In light of this reflection, write a prayer from your heart to God's heart.

_____

_____

_____

_____

_____

_____

_____

_____

Lord, help me to give my best—my all—for You. Guide me to use the gifts
and talents You've given me for Your glory. In Jesus' name, amen.

Notes

1. Christin Ditchfield, *A Way with Words: What Women Should Know About the Power They Possess* (Wheaton, IL: Crossway Books, 2010), pp. 158-159.
2. Thomas à Kempis (1380-1471), from The Imitation of Christ.
3. Lysa TerKeurst, *Radically Obedient, Radically Blessed: Experiencing God in Extraordinary Ways* (Eugene, OR: Harvest House Publishers, 2003), p. 37.
4. Ditchfield, *A Way with Words,* pp. 161-162.

Group Prayer Requests

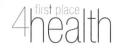

Today's Date: _____

Name	Request

Results

_____

_____

_____

_____

_____

_____

growing in grace

When you stop and think about it, many of our Bible heroes—the great men and women of the faith—did not begin so heroically. They were a bunch of messed-up, mixed-up people! Abraham was a coward. Jacob was a liar. Moses was a hothead. Rahab was a prostitute. David was an adulterer. Jonah was a whiner. Matthew was a cheater. Peter was a blowhard. Martha was a busybody. Thomas was a doubter. Prior to his conversion, the apostle Paul was a Pharisee who killed Christians in the name of God.

These men and women were all too human. They had serious character flaws. They made major mistakes. But they served an awesome God. An amazing God. A God, who in His amazing grace, forgave them. A God who redeemed them and restored them (see Romans 3:23-24).

In Ephesians 1:6-7, Paul writes, "So we praise God for the glorious grace he has poured out on us who belong to his dear Son. He is so rich in kindness and grace that he purchased our freedom with the blood of his Son and forgave our sins" (*NLT*). By God's grace, He worked in and through these men and women—these very flawed and frail human beings—to accomplish great and mighty things for His kingdom. By this same grace, He has worked in *us* and through *us* to accomplish great and mighty things for His kingdom.

How amazing! What a blessing! May each one of us receive God's grace and walk in it—grow in it—today.

WHAT GRACE IS

*Lord, teach me to understand what Your grace is all about. Help me
to believe it and receive it in Jesus' name, amen.*

Let's look at our memory verse, John 1:16, in context. John 1:14 tells us
that "the Word became flesh and made his dwelling among us." How
does this verse go on to describe Jesus?

_____

_____

_____

Read John 1:16-17. From where do our blessings spring? What is their
source?

_____

_____

_____

What did Moses give us (see verse 17)?

_____

_____

_____

Remember that the apostle Paul said that the Law was meant to help us
see our sinfulness—in our inability to follow it—so that we would recognize our need for a Savior. According to John 1:17, what has come to us
through Jesus?

_____

_____

_____

"Grace" as it is used in Scripture can be defined as "love and kindness
shown to someone who does not deserve it—especially the forgiveness
God shows to us."[1] God showed grace to all people by sending His Son,

Jesus, to be our Savior, and through His grace He allows us to become members of His family. No one can earn God's *grace* by trying to be good; it is a free gift from God. Turn to Romans 5:1-5.

Complete the following sentences about the things God's grace has done for us, given us or made it possible for us to do:

By God's grace, we have been _____

We have been given _____

Believing in Jesus gives us access to the grace in which _____

Because of God's grace we can _____

We can also _____

God's grace produces in us _____

Reflecting on the word "grace," author Philip Yancey wrote that "grace is indeed amazing. . . . It contains the essence of the gospel as a drop of water can contain the image of the sun."[2] In your own words, describe what God's grace means to you personally and why it is so amazing in your life. (If you need help, read Romans 5:6-8.)

_____

_____

_____

Thank You, Jesus, for allowing me to experience the fullness of Your grace.
Help me to recognize all that You have to give me. Amen.

SAVING GRACE
Day 2

Thank You, Jesus, that Your grace is greater than all my sin! Amen.

Read Ephesians 2:1-10. According to this passage, why did God save us (see verses 4,7)?

_____

_____

_____

We know that we cannot earn our salvation by doing good works (see verses 8-9). So why then do we do good works (see verse 10)?

_____

_____

_____

Turn to James 4:6,10. What happens when we struggle, when we stumble, when we fall and fail?

_____

_____

_____

God doesn't mock us. He doesn't judge us. He doesn't criticize or condemn us. He helps us! Read Romans 8:1. What is God's attitude toward us when we have His gift of grace?

_____

_____

_____

Often we feel so miserable about our failures and mistakes. We feel so guilty. We try to hide from God—like Adam and Eve—which only makes us feel worse. And we begin a downward spiral that leads to greater sin, greater guilt and greater despair. When this happens, what do we need to remember, according to Ephesians 1:7?

_____

_____

_____

What should we do when we find ourselves making poor choices, giving in to temptation and sin (see James 4:7)?

_____

_____

_____

Oswald Chambers noted, "I must realize that my obedience even in the smallest detail of life has all of the omnipotent power of the grace of God behind it. If I will do my duty, not for duty's sake, but because I believe God is engineering my circumstances, then at the very point of my obedience, all of the magnificent grace of God is mine through the glorious atonement by the Cross of Christ."[3] When we yield our lives to God and rely on His grace, He gives us the strength to resist temptation.

Father, thank You that You have given me the grace to resist temptation and to get back up when I've given in to it. Help me stand firm. Amen.

WHAT GRACE CAN DO Day 3

Lord, there is so much more to Your grace than I can begin to understand or imagine. Help me to see how Your grace is at work in my life today. Amen.

In 2 Peter 3:18, we are instructed to "grow in the grace and knowledge of our Lord and Savior Jesus Christ." According to the following Scriptures, what does it mean to grow in grace, and what can God's grace do in us and through us?

2 Corinthians 9:8

_____

_____

_____

2 Thessalonians 2:16-17

_____

_____

_____

Titus 2:11-14

_____

_____

_____

Take a moment to think about your First Place 4 Health journey. Think of the goals that you've set, the commitments that you've made, the things you know that God has asked you to do. Now choose two or three of these items and write them as statements of faith that you will be able to accomplish them by God's grace.

By God's grace, I will _____

_____

By God's grace, I will _____

_____

By God's grace, I will _____

_____

Lord, I realize I can accomplish nothing without Your grace to change me from the inside out, to motivate and inspire me, to help me and strengthen me. Please give me all that I need today. Amen.

Day 4 — RECEIVING GOD'S GRACE

Jesus, thank You for pouring Your mercy and grace on my life today. I receive it joyfully, with thanksgiving in my heart! Your grace is amazing! Amen.

Let's look at an example from the Bible that vividly shows us what it means to experience God's grace. Read Jonah 1:1-17. God called Jonah to go and preach to the people of Nineveh, but how did Jonah respond (see verse 3)?

_____

_____

_____

How did God get Jonah's attention (see verses 4,17)?

_____

_____

_____

Note that in His mercy and grace, God did not strike Jonah dead for his disobedience. He didn't abandon Jonah or turn His back on him. Instead, He pursued him. God went after His wayward, disobedient child. He brought him to a place of humiliation, a place of desperation, a place of salvation. Read Jonah 2:1-10. Where was Jonah when he offered this heartfelt prayer (see verse 1)?

When Jonah was confronted with his sinfulness, his wretchedness, his helplessness, what did he do (see verse 7)?

What did Jonah learn from this experience (see verses 8-9)?

To what "idols" might Jonah have been clinging? (Note that an idol is anything that takes the place of God in our hearts, anything we turn to instead of Him, or anything that rivals Him for our attention, affection and devotion.)

To what kinds of idols do many people cling today?

_____

_____

_____

What does this cost that person (see verse 8)?

_____

_____

_____

According to Jonah, what is the better way (see verse 9)?

_____

_____

_____

Jonah wasn't the only one to experience God's grace in this story. Who else received the grace of God through Jonah's testimony (see Jonah 1:16; 3:10)?

_____

_____

_____

_____

Lord, help me to let go of any idols that would steal my heart away from You. Let my life be a testimony to Your amazing grace today. Amen.

Day
5

EXTENDING GOD'S GRACE

Father, You are so kind, so compassionate, so merciful toward all You have made. I praise Your holy name! Amen.

Many Bible stories have a Part Two, and the story of Jonah is no exception. The runaway prophet had experienced God's grace in a spectacular, miraculous, life-changing way. He became one of the most successful prophets in the Bible. The people of Nineveh actually listened to him, instead of stoning him to death or sawing him in half. More than that, they repented of their sin—all of them—the king and everyone else. You would think Jonah would have been thrilled with the results, but this was not the case.

Read Jonah 4:1-3. How did Jonah respond to seeing God's mercy and grace—the same mercy and grace that he himself had received—extended to the people of Nineveh?

_____

_____

_____

_____

Jonah actually had the nerve to be angry with God for forgiving the people of Nineveh. He complained about God being so "gracious and compassionate . . . slow to anger and abounding in love" (verse 2). It seems that he wanted to see those wicked people get what they deserved. Perhaps he forgot that if God had taken that attitude with him, he would still be inside the fish. God forgave Jonah when he repented, but Jonah was outraged when God forgave the people of Nineveh when they repented.

Are we impatient or exasperated with those who can't seem to get their act together? Are we ever eager to see other people suffer the consequences of their actions? Do we sometimes pray that they'll repent, yet we secretly hope they'll get what they deserve? Read the parable Jesus told about the unmerciful servant in Matthew 18:23-35. A man owed his king an enormous debt that he could not hope to repay. How did the king respond to his cry for mercy (see verse 27)?

_____

_____

_____

_____

Another man owed the first man a much smaller debt. How did the first man respond to the second man's cry for mercy (see verse 30)?

_____

_____

_____

_____

What is the moral of the story?

_____

_____

_____

Read Luke 6:36-37. What character traits should we exhibit?

_____

_____

_____

_____

What traits should we avoid?

_____

_____

_____

_____

Father, help me to be merciful as You are merciful, to share freely the grace I have received from You. Keep my heart tender toward others. Amen.

Day 6

REFLECTION AND APPLICATION

Lord, in You there is forgiveness, mercy and grace. No sin is too great to be covered by Your precious blood. Amen.

In John 8:1-11, the apostle John described a powerful scene in which Jesus was confronted by the Pharisees and teachers of the law. They brought to Jesus a woman caught in adultery, and they reminded Him that the Law of Moses says she should be stoned to death. When they asked Jesus what He thought of the matter, He replied simply, "Let him who is without sin cast the first stone." Then the Scripture says, "Those who heard began to go away one at a time, the older ones first."

"The older ones first." Did you notice that? Why did the older ones leave first? Perhaps it's because the older we get, the more experience we have in the battles of the flesh. When we're young—physically and spiritually—we're full of enthusiasm and zeal and arrogance. We're caught up in the pride of youth, confident in our own strength and intolerant of others' weaknesses.

But those who have matured—in years and in faith—have come to realize just how weak and frail the human flesh really is, the depths to which our sin nature will sink. We understand the struggles and the frustrations. We've been repeatedly humbled by our own failures, so we learn not to be so quick to condemn others. There but for the grace of God . . .

"Let him who is without sin cast the first stone." Jesus brought the Pharisees up short when He reminded them of this truth. They were convicted of the sinfulness of their own hearts. They knew that they had no right to condemn anyone else. So they dropped their stones and went away. May God grant us the wisdom and humility and grace to do the same.

Today, spend a few moments in quiet reflection. Ask God to show you if there are those in your life toward whom your heart has been hard, unmerciful or unforgiving—people you have judged, criticized or condemned. Write their names down, and next to each name, tell how you will extend grace to him or her. Respond as the Holy Spirit leads you.

_____

_____

_____

_____

_____

Lord, help me never to forget how much I need Your mercy and grace in my life. Let me be eager to extend that grace to others. In Jesus' name, amen.

REFLECTION AND APPLICATION

Jesus, I know I don't deserve Your mercy and grace, but I'm so grateful for it. Help me to grow in Your grace today. Amen.

Look again at the scene John describes about the woman caught in adultery in John 8:1-11. Once Jesus had dealt with the Pharisees, He turned and spoke to the woman. He asked her if anyone had condemned her—if anyone had pronounced judgment on her. She answered, "No one, sir." Jesus then said to her, "Then neither do I condemn you." What did He tell her to do (see verse 11)?

_____

_____

_____

_____

_____

In some Bible translations (the *New Living Translation*, for example), this verse reads, "Go and sin no more." The ulterior motives of the Pharisees do not negate the fact that the woman was, in fact, guilty of the sin of which she had been accused. She knew it, and Jesus knew it. But Jesus declared her not guilty. In His love, His mercy and His grace, He chose to forgive her. In the same way, He chooses to forgive each of us. Reflect on some of the things for which you have been forgiven. Do you still feel guilty about them? Do you truly believe that you have been forgiven? Why or why not?

_____

_____

_____

_____

_____

Does God's grace and forgiveness mean that your sin doesn't matter to God, that you can go on sinning without giving it another thought (see

Romans 6:1-4)? What is the outward sign of the grace we receive inside when we believe in Jesus?

_____

_____

_____

_____

_____

How should we respond to the grace of God? How will you respond today?

_____

_____

_____

_____

Lord, I thank You with all my heart for Your forgiveness, mercy and grace. Help me to leave my life of sin and live the new life that You have given me. In Jesus' precious name, amen.

Notes

1. Henrietta Mears, *What the Bible Is All About* (Ventura, CA: Regal Books, 1998), p. 695.
2. Philip Yancey, *What's So Amazing About Grace* (Grand Rapids, MI: Zondervan, 1997), p. 13.
3. Oswald Chambers, *My Utmost for His Highest,* special updated ed., ed. James Reimann (Grand Rapids, MI: Discovery House Publishers, 1995), June 15.

Group Prayer Requests

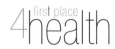

Today's Date: _____

Name	Request

Results

_____

_____

_____

_____

_____

surrendering to
His lordship

SCRIPTURE MEMORY VERSE
*That at the name of Jesus every knee should bow, in heaven
and on earth and under the earth, and every tongue confess
that Jesus Christ is Lord, to the glory of God the Father.*
PHILIPPIANS 2:10-11

When he was exiled to the island of St. Helena, French emperor Napoleon Bonaparte had a lot of time to reflect on a great many things. One day, he called a friend to his side and asked him, "Can you tell me who Jesus Christ was?" The friend politely declined to respond. So Napoleon said to him:

> Well then, I will tell you. Alexander, Caesar, Charlemagne, and I myself have founded great empires; but upon what did these creations of our genius depend? Upon force. Jesus alone founded His empire upon love, and to this very day millions will die for Him. . . . I think I understand something of human nature; and I tell you, all these were men, and I am a man: none else is like Him; Jesus Christ was more than a man . . . I have inspired multitudes with such an enthusiastic devotion that they would have died for me . . . but to do this it was necessary that I should be visibly present with the electric influence of my looks, my words, of my voice. When I saw men and spoke to them, I lighted up the flame of self-devotion in their hearts. . . .

Christ alone has succeeded in so raising the mind of man toward the unseen, that it becomes insensitive to the barriers of time and space. Across a chasm of eighteen hundred years, Jesus Christ makes a demand which is beyond all others difficult to satisfy; He asks for that which a philosopher may often seek in vain at the hands of his friends, or a father of his children, or a bride of her spouse, or a man of his brother. He asks for the human heart; He will have it entirely to Himself. He demands it unconditionally; and forthwith His demand is granted. Wonderful! In defiance of time and space, the soul of man, with all its powers and faculties, becomes an annexation to the empire of Christ.

All who sincerely believe in Him, experience that remarkable, supernatural love toward Him. This phenomenon is unaccountable; it is altogether beyond the scope of man's creative powers. Time, the great destroyer, is powerless to extinguish this sacred flame; time can neither exhaust its strength nor put a limit to its range. This is it, which strikes me most; I have often thought of it. This it is which proves to me quite convincingly the Divinity of Jesus Christ.[1]

There is no one like Jesus. No human can demand and command as Jesus did and does, and everyone who submits to His lordship will have an eternal life. One day, all will recognize and confess that Jesus is Lord.

Day 1 LORDSHIP

Jesus, truly You are the Son of God, the risen Savior—my Savior and my friend. I owe all my love and devotion to You. Amen.

It's been said that when it comes to Jesus, there are three groups of people: (1) those who neither call Him Lord nor do the things that He says; (2) those who call Him Lord but do not do the things that He says; and

(3) those who call Him Lord and do the things that He says. In which group of people do you find yourself today?

_____

_____

_____

_____

Some people say that Jesus was a great moral teacher, but they deny that He was and is the Son of God. Instead, they profess to respect Him as a great moral teacher. However, when you look at the things Jesus said—the claims He made about Himself in Scripture—this position becomes untenable. As C. S. Lewis once noted:

> A man who was merely a man and said the sort of things Jesus said would not be a great moral teacher. He would either be a lunatic—on a level with the man who says he is a poached egg—or else he would be the Devil of Hell. You must make your choice. Either this man was, and is, the Son of God: or else a madman or something worse. You can shut Him up for a fool, you can spit at Him and kill Him as a demon; or you can fall at His feet and call Him Lord and God. But let us not come with any patronizing nonsense about His being a great moral teacher. He has not left that open to us. He did not intend to. Now it seems to me obvious that He was neither a lunatic nor a fiend: and consequently, however strange or terrifying or unlikely it may seem, I have to accept the view that He was and is God.[2]

Some people believe that Jesus is the Son of God. Many call Him their Savior. But how many would call Him "Lord"? As Napoleon pointed out, Jesus demands that we unconditionally hand our hearts to Him and submit to His absolute claim to our devotion, our obedience and our allegiance. According to the following Scriptures, why does Jesus have the right to claim these things?

Revelation 4:11

_____
_____
_____
_____

Revelation 5:9

_____
_____
_____
_____

Revelation 19:11-16

_____
_____
_____
_____

_Lord Jesus, You are worthy of all my love, all my trust, all my obedience. I
live to bring You glory and to worship Your precious and holy name. Amen._

Day 2   **SUBMISSION**

_Father, teach me to be more like Jesus. Mold me and make me into the image
of Your precious Son. To Him be the glory, now and forever! Amen._

Read Philippians 2:5-11. Why did God exalt Jesus and give Him "the
name above all names" (see verse 8)?

_____
_____
_____
_____
_____

According to John 6:38, why did Jesus come to earth?

_____

_____

_____

_____

Turn to Matthew 26:36-46. What did Jesus pray in the Garden of Gethsemane (see verses 39,42,44)?

_____

_____

_____

_____

Why did Jesus have to suffer and die on the cross (see Hebrews 5:8-9)?

_____

_____

_____

_____

Jesus surrendered Himself completely to the will of His Father. He set an example for us of perfect obedience, perfect submission, perfect surrender. In Ephesians 5:1-2, how does Paul urge us to respond?

_____

_____

_____

_____

According to Romans 12:1-2, what will we learn if we do?

_____

_____

_____

_____

According to the following Scriptures, why is it important to know the will of God?

Matthew 7:21

_____
_____
_____
_____
_____

Colossians 1:9-10

_____
_____
_____
_____
_____

1 John 2:17

_____
_____
_____
_____
_____

1 John 5:14-15

_____
_____
_____
_____
_____

Lord, may Your will be done on earth—and in my life—as it is in heaven, perfectly and completely. In Jesus' name, amen.

OBEDIENCE

Thank You, Jesus, for Your redeeming love. Help me to live a life worthy of the gospel—one that honors You and the sacrifice You made for me. Amen.

Look up Galatians 2:20. How is a person "crucified with Christ"?

_____

_____

_____

_____

Read Psalm 40:8. When the Word of God (Jesus) lives in us, what will we desire?

_____

_____

_____

_____

Read John 4:1-42. This passage describes a time when Jesus spent His day reaching out to a woman at a well and later all of her friends and family, as well as the local townspeople. He was drawing them to Himself—to a life-changing love relationship with Him. What was uppermost on the minds of His disciples (see verse 31)?

_____

_____

_____

_____

From where did Jesus draw His nourishment? What gave Him a sense of satisfaction and fulfillment? What gave Him strength (see verse 34)?

_____

_____

_____

_____

When Jesus is not Lord of our hearts and lives, we tend to turn to other things, other people and other places to meet our spiritual, physical and emotional needs. We only do God's will—what He has asked us to do—when it is convenient for us or when it lines up with our will. This is not acceptable to Jesus. In Luke 6:46, He asked His disciples, "Why do you call me, 'Lord, Lord,' and do not do what I say?" What are some of the things that you know are God's will for you right now?

_____

_____

_____

_____

Are you doing these things? Why or why not?

_____

_____

_____

_____

In light of your answer, what does this tell you about the position that Christ has in your life today?

_____

_____

_____

_____

If there are things of which you are uncertain—if you have questions about God's will in certain circumstances or situations—ask Him to reveal His will to you and give you clear direction in these things. He promises that He will give you what you need, if you ask.

Lord, show me Your will and help me to walk in it. Strengthen me by Your Spirit as I obey Your Word. Amen.

REBELLION

Lord Jesus, Your Name is above every name, Your power above all power.
You are the King of kings and Lord of lords. My life belongs to You. Amen.

In the Old Testament, God delivered the Israelites from slavery in Egypt and led them across the desert to a land He had promised to give them. It was a fruitful land, flowing "with milk and honey" (Numbers 13:27). It also had some pretty fierce inhabitants already living there. But God told His people not to be afraid.

Read Exodus 6:6-8. What had God promised to do for the Israelites?

_____

_____

_____

_____

Read Numbers 13:3–14:4. How did the people respond when they reached the Promised Land (see verse 32)?

_____

_____

_____

_____

C. S. Lewis wrote, "There are two kinds of people: those who say to God, 'Thy will be done,' and those to whom God says, 'All right, then, have it your way.' "[3] This was certainly the case with the Israelites. They listened to fear and doubt and flat-out refused to enter the Promised Land as God had commanded them. According to Numbers 14:20-23, how did God respond to the peoples' rebellion?

_____

_____

_____

_____

The Israelites would have to wander in the desert until every member of their generation had died. Then their children would inherit the Promised Land. When the people realized what they had lost—the cost of their disobedience—they did an abrupt about-face. They decided they would obey God, but it was too late. They tried to enter the Promised Land on their own (without God's blessing or protection), and they were defeated in battle. They had to return to the desert. To what is rebellion and arrogance— ego and stubborn self-will—compared in the Bible (see 1 Samuel 15:23)?

_____

_____

_____

_____

When you give way to a proud and rebellious spirit, you set yourself up in God's place. You're worshiping your own god—you! The prophet Isaiah points out how foolish it is to resist and rebel against God:

> "What sorrow awaits those who argue with their Creator. Does a clay pot argue with its maker? Does the clay dispute with the one who shapes it, saying, 'Stop, you're doing it wrong!' Does the pot exclaim, 'How clumsy can you be?' " . . . This is what the LORD says—the Holy One of Israel and your Creator: "Do you question what I do for my children? Do you give me orders about the work of my hands? I am the one who made the earth and created people to live on it. With my hands I stretched out the heavens. All the stars are at my command" (Isaiah 45:9-12, _NLT_).

Ask God to show you if there's any area of your heart or life in which you've been disobeying Him, arguing with Him or rebelling against Him. Ask Him to forgive you and make you willing to obey (see Psalm 51).

Lord, don't let me harden my heart toward You. Help me to hear and obey. In Jesus' name, amen.

ABANDONMENT Day 5

Lord, Your love is better than life. I will praise You with all my heart for as long as I live! Amen.

Read Matthew 16:24. If we want to walk with Jesus, what must we be willing to do?

_____

_____

_____

_____

A similar verse appears in Luke 9:23. What important word is added?

_____

_____

_____

_____

Do you wrestle with any reluctance to abandon, or surrender, yourself completely to Jesus? If so, why?

_____

_____

_____

_____

_____

As Oswald Chambers once noted, "We will never know the joy of self-sacrifice until we surrender in every detail of our lives. Yet self-surrender is the most difficult thing for us to do. . . . But as soon as we do totally surrender, abandoning ourselves to Jesus, the Holy Spirit gives us a taste of His joy. . . . When the Holy Spirit comes into our lives, our greatest desire is to lay down our lives for Jesus. Yet the thought of self-sacrifice never even crosses our minds, because sacrifice is the Holy Spirit's ultimate expression of love."[4] Read Revelation 12:10-11. The believers described in this passage were fearless in facing down the enemy of their souls. For what in particular does the verse praise them?

_____

_____

_____

As martyred missionary Jim Elliot famously said, "He is no fool who gives what he cannot keep to gain that which he cannot lose." Few of us will be asked to lay down our lives for the gospel. By comparison, the sacrifices God asks most of us to make are relatively small. What sacrifices do you regard as easy to make?

_____

_____

_____

What sacrifices do you regard as things that you *have to* make?

_____

_____

_____

You can *choose* to make all of your sacrifices with a joyful heart, out of love for Jesus, totally abandoning yourself to His everlasting love.

> *Lord, help me to love You with reckless abandon, being willing to give all that I have and all that I am to You! Amen.*

Day 6 REFLECTION AND APPLICATION

God, I know that You know what You're doing in my life, even when I don't. Help me to trust You and surrender myself to You completely. Amen.

Some of us feel as if we've made a mess of our lives. We haven't lived the way we should. We've made mistakes and poor choices. It's true that we've repented and asked God for forgiveness. But deep down inside, we're sometimes tempted to feel a sense of hopelessness and despair. We wonder if it might be too late—if our lives may be ruined beyond repair.

In Jeremiah 18:1-6, the Lord instructed the prophet to go down to the potter's house, where He would deliver His message. When Jeremiah went there, he saw the potter working at the wheel. But the clay the man was making was misshapen, so the potter formed it into another pot, shaping it the way that seemed best to him. Then the Lord said to Jeremiah, "O house of Israel, can I not do with you as this potter does? . . . Like clay in the hand of the potter, so are you in my hand" (Jeremiah 18:1-6).

So great is the tender mercy of our God that regardless of our past failures, in spite of our present weakness, He *can* and *will* use us for His glory—as long as we're fully surrendered to Him.

In what ways do you, like Israel, need to be reformed by the Potter?

_____

_____

_____

In what ways, if any, are you resisting that change in your life? What are your fears and concerns when you think of God remolding your life?

_____

_____

_____

What would be the benefits to you personally of allowing God to do that work in your situation?

_____

_____

_____

Remember not to get impatient and start climbing off the potter's wheel. Don't forget that it's not up to us to determine the shape or the design. Let God do what He does best. Trust Him to complete the work that He's already begun in your heart and life. Remember that He makes all things beautiful in His time (see Ecclesiastes 3:11).

Lord, help me to be patient with the process and allow You to mold me and make me into the person You created me to be. I trust You, even when I don't understand. Amen.

Day 7

REFLECTION AND APPLICATION

Jesus, You are my Lord and Savior. Help me to give myself completely to You. Be glorified in my life today. Amen.

Look up Isaiah 64:8 and put it in your own words in the space provided below.

_____

_____

_____

_____

Underline any words or phrases from this hymn, "Have Thine Own Way, Lord," that speak to your heart today:

Have Thine own way, Lord! Have Thine own way!
Thou art the Potter, I am the clay.
Mold me and make me after Thy will,
While I am waiting, yielded and still.

Have Thine own way, Lord! Have Thine own way!
Search me and try me, Master, today!
Whiter than snow, Lord, wash me just now,
As in Thy presence humbly I bow.

Have Thine own way, Lord! Have Thine own way!
Wounded and weary, help me, I pray!
Power, all power, surely is Thine!
Touch me and heal me, Savior divine.

Have Thine own way, Lord! Have Thine own way!
Hold o'er my being absolute sway!
Fill with Thy Spirit 'till all shall see
Christ only, always, living in me.[5]

This hymn describes what it means to say that Jesus is Lord. If you are willing to give yourself to Him fully and completely, write a prayer of surrender in the space below. If you're not there yet, but you're willing to be made willing, then put that in this prayer from your heart to God's heart.

_____

_____

_____

_____

Lord, I want to worship You with all my heart, with all my soul and with all my strength (see Deuteronomy 6:5). Everything I have, everything I am and ever hope to be, help me to surrender to You—now and forever. Amen.

Notes

1. Napoleon Bonaparte, quoted in Ravi Zacharias, *Jesus Among Other Gods* (Nashville, TN: Word Publishing Group, 2000), pp. 148-50.
2. C. S. Lewis, *Mere Christianity* (London: Harper Collins, 1954), pp. 54,56.
3. C.S. Lewis, *The Screwtape Letters* (San Francisco: Harper Collins, 2005).
4. Oswald Chambers, *My Utmost for His Highest*, ed. James Reimann (Grand Rapids, MI: Discovery House Publishers, 1995), August 25.
5. Adelaide A. Pollard (1862-1934), "Have Thine Own Way, Lord." Cyberhymnal.org. November 9, 2007. http://www.cyberhymnal.org/htm/h/t/hthineow.htm.

Group Prayer Requests

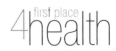

Today's Date: _____

Name	Request

Results

_____

_____

_____

_____

_____

Week Ten

standing
by faith

SCRIPTURE MEMORY VERSE
*No one will be able to stand up against you all the days of your life. As I was
with Moses, so I will be with you; I will never leave you nor forsake you.*
JOSHUA 1:5

Have you ever been forgotten? When you were a child, did your parents
ever accidentally leave you at a store, a gas station or a restaurant? Was
there ever a time when each parent thought the other one had picked
you up from school? Were you ever left off the invitation list to a special
party? Have you ever been ignored by others in a social setting, at church
or at work?

There's no question that at some point or another, we've all experienced the pain of feeling alone, abandoned, neglected or unloved—times
when even God seemed very far away. The Old Testament describes an oc-
casion when God's people experienced that same kind of pain. Isaiah
49:14-15 tells us, "Zion said, 'The LORD has forsaken me, and my Lord has
forgotten me.'" But God answered them, "Can a woman forget her nurs-
ing child, and not have compassion on the son of her womb?" (*NKJV*). Not
likely! God continued, "They may forget. Yet I will not forget you. See, I
have inscribed you on the palms of My hands" (Isaiah 49:15-16, *NKJV*).

Think about that a moment: *God has inscribed us on the palms of His
hands.* Some Bible versions have translated "inscribed" as "engraved,"
"tattooed" or "indelibly imprinted." What a powerful picture of the
steadfast love the Lord has for us. Others may forget us or ignore us or

leave us off their lists. Others may forsake us or abandon us. But our heavenly Father never will. Because of His love for us, we are never forsaken. We are never forgotten.

In the New Testament, Jesus gave us this precious promise: "Lo, I am with you always, even to the end of the age" (Matthew 28:20, *NKJV*). Let these words bring comfort and assurance to your heart today as you stand by faith on the truth of God's Word.[1]

Day 1 — GOD IS MIGHTY

Lord, You are my rock, my fortress and my deliverer. Because of You, I know I have nothing to fear. Amen.

As Joshua prepared to lead a new generation of God's people into the Promised Land, he faced an incredibly difficult task: following in the footsteps of a spiritual giant like Moses and trying to lead a notoriously rebellious and disobedient people. The land itself was filled with pagan peoples—some of them giants—that Joshua and his army would have to drive out. No doubt, the Lord's words of encouragement, recorded in this week's memory verse, were just what Joshua desperately needed to hear.

Read Joshua 1:9. What else did God say to Joshua?

_____

_____

_____

_____

What "giants" are you facing in your life today? What trials or temptations? What difficult—even impossible—people or circumstances?

_____

_____

_____

_____

Look up Isaiah 54:16-17. How is the sovereignty of God described (see verse 16)?

_____

_____

_____

_____

God has created all things, including the blacksmith who forges weapons of destruction and the men who use such weapons. This is true in a literal sense, but it is also true in a spiritual sense, in that "the destroyer" also refers to, as someone once put it, "God's devil!" He's on a short leash. He can only do what God allows him to do. According to verse 17, what two things does God promise?

_____

_____

_____

_____

Why does He do this for us (see verse 17)?

_____

_____

_____

_____

Read Psalm 18:32-34. What else does God do for us?

_____

_____

_____

_____

God's blessings allow us to thrive, just as they helped David, the author of this psalm, to thrive. Which of these blessings are you in special need of today? Why?

_____

_____

_____

_____

Father, thank You that You don't send me into battle alone and unprepared. You go before me, and You make sure I have everything I need. Amen.

Day 2

GOD IS FAITHFUL

Lord Jesus, thank You that You are always true to Your Word. You keep Your promises and You protect Your own. Amen.

Read Lamentations 3:22-23. Why is it that God's love and compassion never fail?

_____

_____

_____

_____

How is God's faithfulness to His promises described (see verse 23)?

_____

_____

_____

_____

What observation does David make in Psalm 37:25?

_____

_____

_____

_____

Why is God faithful (see Psalm 37:28)?

_____

_____

_____

_____

_____

Read Psalm 27. In this psalm, David expresses his confidence that God is faithful and will keep His promises, so David will wait for what he is sure will happen, even though he can't see it. In effect, David will faithfully wait for God's faithfulness to manifest itself. What declaration does David make in Psalm 27:13?

_____

_____

_____

_____

_____

Look up 1 Thessalonians 5:23-24. Why does Paul say he has confidence in God?

_____

_____

_____

_____

_____

There's another way that God expressed His faithfulness. Read 1 Corinthians 1:8-9. What does the apostle Paul promise that God will do?

_____

_____

_____

_____

_____

Why should you feel confident in God's faithfulness to help you on your First Place 4 Health journey?

_____

_____

_____

_____

Lord Jesus, You are faithful to keep Your promises. Help me to stay confident in You and to stay strong until the end. In Your precious name, amen.

Day 3 GOD IS CONSTANT

Lord, You are the one constant in my life—my rock, my refuge, my redeemer. I run to You! Amen.

Look up Hebrews 13:5-8. These verses echo this week's memory verse. God will never leave us or forsake us, and no one can harm us. We can draw both comfort and courage from reflecting on the lives of those who have walked with God before us (like Moses), and we can and should imitate their faith. What other important statement does this passage make (see verse 8)?

_____

_____

_____

Yesterday we talked about God's faithfulness. Today we're looking at His constancy. In our culture, we love to hear about things that are "new and improved" or the "latest and greatest." When we describe something as the "same old, same old," it's usually a bad thing. So why should we be so eternally grateful that God is always the same—that He's constant and steadfast? Well, think about what the opposite would be: fickle, capricious, temperamental, unstable, unsteady, unreliable.

So when God says (as He does in Malachi 3:6), "I, the LORD, do not change," that's a wonderful thing. He is just as good, just as loving, just as merciful, just as kind as He has always been. And just as powerful. Think about that. The same God who created the heavens and the earth, parted the Red Sea, demolished the walls of Jericho, walked on water and rose from the dead is the same One who watches over you and me.

What does James 1:17 say about God?

_____

_____

_____

_____

Look up what the apostle Paul refers to as "a trustworthy saying" in 2 Timothy 2:11-13. What will happen to us if we die to our old selves and put our faith in Jesus (see verse 11)?

_____

_____

_____

_____

What will happen if we put up with hardships (see verse 12)?

_____

_____

_____

_____

What will happen if we give up on Jesus or don't follow His commands—if we're "faithless" (verse 13)?

_____

_____

_____

_____

We can choose to walk away from God, to reject Him. And if we do, there will be consequences: God will reject (or disown) us. But nothing we do will cause Him to behave badly—to go back on His Word or betray His own character and integrity. God cannot be unfaithful to us, even when we are unfaithful to Him, because it simply isn't in His nature. He remains true to who He is because that's who He is. Look up Deuteronomy 32:3-4. Why should we praise the greatness of our God?

_____

_____

_____

_____

How is this (or why should this be) a comforting or encouraging thought?

_____

_____

_____

_____

*God, thank You that You are not only faithful but also constant—
always just, good, kind and merciful. Help me to stay steadfast in my
love for and obedience to You. Amen.*

Day 4

GOD IS PRESENT

*Lord Jesus, what a comfort it is to know that You are always with me—You
surround me with Your love, mercy and grace.*

Read Psalm 46:1. How does this verse describe God?

_____

_____

_____

_____

Now turn to Isaiah 43:1-3. According to these verses, why shouldn't we be afraid (see verse 1)?

_____

_____

_____

_____

_____

Where will God be when we go through trials and temptations (see verses 2-3)?

_____

_____

_____

_____

_____

Shadrach, Meshach and Abednego experienced the truth of this precious promise. In Daniel 3:4-6, what did the king of Babylon command the people to do?

_____

_____

_____

_____

_____

How did Shadrach, Meshach and Abednego respond to the king's threats against them (see Daniel 3:16-18)?

_____

_____

_____

_____

_____

The king made good on his threats. Where was God when His servants were thrown into the fiery furnace (see verse 25)?

_____

_____

_____

_____

Where is God when you face obstacles and challenges and trials and tribulations? Where is He when life hurts, when it seems like your world is falling apart?

_____

_____

_____

_____

We don't always emerge from the heat of the battle unscathed—at least not in an earthly sense. Sometimes we do get wounded. We carry battle scars. Jacob wrestled with God and forever after walked with a limp (see Genesis 32:22-32). But in a spiritual sense, in an eternal sense, there is nothing that the enemy of our souls can do to us. There is nothing he can take from us. If we live, God is with us. If we die, we are with God. He is always present. And He is always actively at work in our hearts and lives and in the hearts and lives of those around us. What does this mean to you personally today?

_____

_____

_____

_____

_____

_Father, never let me forget that I don't have to face everything—
or anything—on my own. You are always with me, and You are
always ready to help me. Amen._

GOD IS VICTORIOUS

Day 5

Jesus, risen Prince of Victory, all Your enemies lie vanquished at Your feet. Hallelujah! Amen.

Read Psalm 24:7-10. Who is the "King of glory," and how is He described?

_____

_____

_____

_____

_____

Look up Deuteronomy 20:3-4. What instructions were given to God's people before they went into battle? What reason did God give as to why the people should follow His instructions?

_____

_____

_____

_____

Turn to Revelation 15:3-4. How is God described?

_____

_____

_____

_____

How will the nations of the earth respond (see verse 4)?

_____

_____

_____

_____

What will happen to Satan (see Revelation 20:10)?

_____

_____

_____

_____

What ultimate victory did Jesus win? Over what did He triumph (see 1 Corinthians 15:53-57)?

_____

_____

_____

_____

In light of this, what advice does the apostle Paul give us (see 1 Corinthians 15:58)?

_____

_____

_____

_____

Why is what you do to accomplish your First Place 4 Health goals "not in vain"?

_____

_____

_____

_____

Almighty God, You alone are worthy of all honor, glory and praise. I rejoice in You and praise Your holy name. I rejoice in Your victory. Amen.

REFLECTION AND APPLICATION

Lord, I'm thankful that You are with me—that I don't have to face anything on my own. You are always with me, and You always answer my call. Amen.

In 2 Chronicles 20, King Jehoshaphat and his tiny nation found themselves in dire circumstances—their enemies had gathered a vast army against them and were soon approaching. The king called the people of Judah to fast and pray. Young and old, men, women and children—they all gathered at the Temple to stand before the Lord.

Jehoshaphat cried out to God, reminding Him of His promise to care for them. He declared the nation's commitment to wait on the Lord for deliverance, and he referred specifically to the crisis at hand—the imminent attack of the enemy. The king concluded his prayer with these simple words: "We do not know what to do, but our eyes are upon you" (2 Chronicles 20:12).

Take a few moments and read Psalm 34. In this psalm, David praises God for answering his prayer to be saved, and he also gives some instructions for following the Lord. What does he tell us in Psalm 34:5?

_____

_____

_____

_____

_____

As Jehoshaphat and his people waited on God, they received this precious promise from Him: "Do not be afraid or discouraged because of this vast army. For the battle is not yours, but God's. . . . Take up your positions; stand firm and see the deliverance the LORD will give you" (2 Chronicles 20:15-17).

Do you ever find yourself overwhelmed by the battles you face? If so, in your prayers for yourself, your loved ones or our nation, you can cry out to God with the words of King Jehoshaphat: "Lord, I don't know what to do, but my eyes are upon You." According to Psalm 34, what assurances do you have that God will always be with you and rescue you in times of trouble—giving you the victory?

_____

In the heat of the battle, Lord, help me to keep my eyes fixed on You.
I know You will fight for me and give me the victory. Amen.

Day 7 — REFLECTION AND APPLICATION

Jesus, You are my Lord and Savior. Help me to give myself completely to You. Be glorified in my life today. Amen.

Let's return to 2 Chronicles 20:21-29 to find out what happened to King Jehoshaphat and the people of Judah. According to this passage, how did God's people march into battle (see verse 21)?

_____

What happened to their enemies (see verses 22-24,29)?

_____

How did the people of Judah respond when it was over (see verses 27-28)?

_____

What should we do when God gives us victory today?

_____

_____

_____

_____

_____

When we want to praise God—to thank Him, pray to Him, worship Him—we can open up the book of Psalms and, just by reading almost any psalm in the book, we will be praising God. In fact, the traditional Hebrew title of the book is *tehillim,* which means "praises."[2] What are some of the reasons you have now to praise God?

_____

_____

_____

_____

_____

In the space below, try your hand at writing a psalm—some words of praise—to God.

_____

_____

_____

_____

_____

Hallelujah! Lord Jesus, You are victorious! All glory and
honor and praise belong to You. Amen.

Notes

1. Christin Ditchfield, *Take It to Heart: Sixty Meditations on God and His Word* (Wheaton, IL: Crossway Books, 2005), pp. 22-23.
2. Kenneth Barker, gen. ed., *The NIV Study Bible* (Grand Rapids, MI: Zondervan Publishing House, 1984), p. 772.

Group Prayer Requests

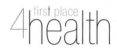

Today's Date: _____

Name	Request

Results

_____

_____

_____

_____

_____

_____

soaring in the strength
of the Spirit

SCRIPTURE MEMORY VERSE

But those who hope in the LORD will renew their strength. They will soar on wings like eagles; they will run and not grow weary, they will walk and not be faint.
ISAIAH 40:31

A pastor shared the following lesson with his congregation that he learned from watching an eagle:

> A couple of years ago, I saw two beautiful bald eagles sitting in the tree in the back corner of our church parking lot. They were being harassed by some obnoxious scrub jays squawking and darting all around them. The two eagles left the tree with a strong flap of their wings and began to circle upwards with calm, powerful strokes. As they moved further skyward, the jays kept at them, but the eagles did not turn toward them and attack, screech, or otherwise defend themselves. They just kept flying higher. Soon the jays could not stay with them. The pesky birds gave up and flew off, leaving the eagles peacefully circling high above.
>
> Today I came upon two eagles on the ground near the pond on our campus. Above their heads, a group of vultures were circling. The eagles didn't like it. They rose up and began to slowly spiral upward from underneath the vultures. With each circle, the eagles pushed the vultures upward until they flew away. Once again, the eagles didn't screech; they didn't attack or try to defend themselves. They just soared higher.

What a great reminder of the truth in Isaiah 40:31: When we calm our hearts before the Lord and focus on Him, we can mount up with the eagle wings of faith and rise up into the throne room of heaven, where we find grace to help us in our time of need.[1]

Isaiah 40:31 in the *Amplified Bible* begins, "Those who wait for the Lord [who expect, look for, and hope in Him]," while the *New Living Translation* states, "But those who trust in the Lord will find new strength." This week, we will look at these words and what they mean for us who long to rise above the trials and temptations of this life and soar on eagles' wings!

Day 1 HOPE

Father, day by day, You renew my strength as I put my hope in You.
Fill me with Your Spirit and help me to rise above the trials I face this week.

Read Isaiah 40:28-31. Whose strength will God renew?

_____

_____

_____

The Hebrew word translated "hope" can also be translated "wait" or "trust." In fact, they often appear together. Turn to Psalm 33:20-22. How does this description of faith connect "hope," "wait" and "trust"?

_____

_____

_____

Look up each of the following verses. According to each, in who or what do we place our hope?

Psalm 31:24 _____

Psalm 33:18 _____

Psalm 130:5 _____

Biblical hope isn't wishful thinking. It's the eager, confident, faith-filled expectancy that God will do as He says, that He will keep His promises, that He will be true to His word. What does Romans 5:6 tell us about this kind of hope?

_____

_____

_____

How can this hope be a source of strength to us today (see 2 Corinthians 3:12; 4:18; Colossians 3:1-4)?

_____

_____

_____

Read Jeremiah 29:11-13. Even during the times when we feel alone and abandoned, why are we still able to hope?

_____

_____

_____

Lord, thank You for the hope that You have given me—the hope that I have in You. Be the strength of my life today. Amen.

WAIT — Day 2

Lord, teach me to be still before You and wait on You for Your direction, Your leading and Your power. Amen.

Sometimes "waiting on the Lord" means being still (see Psalm 46:10). Sometimes it means being patient (see Psalm 37:7). Look up Psalm 27:14. What does the psalmist urge us to do?

_____

_____

_____

Waiting on the Lord means allowing Him to do the work He wants to do in our hearts and lives—letting Him lead us on this journey, without running out ahead of Him or trying to find shortcuts or easier paths. It means that we are not rushing, not pushing and not striving, but trusting in His perfect timing. Note that biblical waiting is not weak and passive and lethargic or unmotivated. On the contrary, it's active, eagerly anticipating the work of God—being intently focused on Him. According to Psalm 33:20-23, why does the psalmist "wait in hope" for the Lord?

_____

_____

_____

_____

For what is he waiting? What does he do while he is waiting (see Psalm 119:166)?

_____

_____

_____

_____

Read Isaiah 26:8. This is part of a song that describes how God's people long for Him to reveal His power and glory as He works in them and through them. What are they doing while they wait?

_____

_____

_____

_____

What are you hoping and trusting in God for today?

_____

_____

_____

_____

What can you do specifically while you wait?

_____

_____

_____

_____

Lord, I'm longing for You, yearning for You, waiting for You.
Help me to walk in obedience to Your Word. Renew my strength and
fill me with Your Spirit. In Jesus' name, amen.

TRUST — Day 3

Lord, You are called "Wonderful, Counselor, Mighty God, Everlasting
Father, Prince of Peace" (Isaiah 9:6). In You I put my trust. Amen.

Look up Psalm 28:7. Why does the psalmist feel like singing?

_____

_____

_____

Now turn to Psalm 9:9-10. According to the psalmist, why should we trust the Lord?

_____

_____

_____

_____

Read Psalm 84:12. How does the psalmist describe those who trust in God?

_____

_____

_____

What assurance do we find in Romans 10:11?

_____

_____

_____

_____

Read Isaiah 25:9. What reward will those who trust in the Lord have?

_____

_____

_____

_____

What was a time when you trusted in God and experienced His mighty power at work in your heart and life?

_____

_____

_____

_____

There are times when, like a bird that has perched on a branch too thin for its weight, we feel as if the branch we're standing on is about to give way. Our world seems to be collapsing—falling out from under us. But there's no reason for us to fear—because on the wings of the Spirit, we can fly!

> Be like a bird that, halting in its flight,
> Rests on a bough too slight.
> And feeling it give way beneath him sings,
> Knowing he hath wings.[2]

By God's grace, we can soar high above the chaos and confusion of our circumstances—with a song of praise on our lips and a peace in our hearts "which surpasses all understanding" (Philippians 4:7, *NKJV*).

When the branches start swaying in the storms of life, don't panic. Trust God. Turn your face to the sky, spread your wings, and fly!

Lord, lift me up and help me soar on the wings of the Spirit. All the glory and honor will be given to You. You are my strength and my song. Amen.

RUN
Day 4

*Lord, in Your strength, I can run and not grow weary.
I can walk and not grow faint. Amen.*

Look up Galatians 6:9 and put it into your own words below. If you like, you can write it as a specific word of encouragement to yourself!

_____

_____

_____

So many people do grow weary in their journey. They do give up, long before they reach the finish. According to this week's memory verse, how do we find the strength to see the race to its end?

_____

_____

_____

Read Psalm 119:32. What did the psalmist find that he could do? Why?

_____

_____

_____

Turn to Hebrews 12:1-3. If we want to "run to win," what do we need to do? (There are at least three things.)

1. _____

2. _____

3. _____

Notice that in this passage from Hebrews, the race that we run is not described as a sprint, a race that is short and fast. We are in a long-distance race, and there are no shortcuts. Fortunately, we have a crowd to cheer us on as we steadily run the course. Who encourages you as you "run" to achieve your First Place 4 Health goals? Who can you encourage?

_____

_____

_____

_____

When you run into obstacles on the "race course," which issues can you address on your own—keeping them just between you and the Lord?

_____

_____

_____

For which issues do you need to involve a trusted friend, family member, a prayer partner or accountability partner?

_____

_____

_____

For which issues would it help to talk to a "coach"—a pastor or Christian counselor?

_____

_____

_____

Determine to do whatever it takes so that you can run with perseverance and receive the reward that God has for you (see 1 Corinthians 9:24-27)!

Lord, help me to throw off everything that hinders and the sin that entangles so I can run with perseverance the race You have marked for me! Amen.

SOAR

*Lord, You teach me to soar on eagles' wings. Thank You for lifting me above
the things that would discourage me. My eyes are fixed on You. Amen.*

According to Zechariah 4:6, how is our victory won?

_____

_____

_____

On whom does God pour out His Spirit (see Acts 2:17-18)?

_____

_____

_____

Turn to Ezekiel 36:25-27. List the things that God promises to do for
His people. (There are at least five.)

1. _____
2. _____
3. _____
4. _____
5. _____

Why will He do this (see verse 27)?

_____

_____

_____

_____

How does 2 Timothy 1:7 describe the spirit that God has given us?

_____

_____

_____

According to Ephesians 1:17, what Spirit did the apostle Paul ask God to give the believers? Why?

_____

_____

_____

Where did Jesus say God's Holy Spirit would live (see John 14:15-17)?

_____

_____

_____

What would the Holy Spirit do (see John 14:26)?

_____

_____

_____

How does this help us "soar" on eagles' wings?

_____

_____

_____

Lord, thank You for giving me Your Holy Spirit to teach me, to guide me and to lead me. I would be lost without You! Amen.

Day 6

REFLECTION AND APPLICATION

God, thank You for speaking into my heart and life, for drawing me into a closer, deeper relationship with You through this journey.

During this study, we've talked about making a fresh start, learning from the past, living in the present, leaning on Jesus and looking ahead to all that He's promised us. We've also talked about giving our best, growing in grace, surrendering to the Lordship of Christ and standing by faith. And this week we talked about what soaring in the strength of the Spirit means.

Now it's time to look back at the things that you have learned in your First Place 4 Health journey. Review each week's study and identify at least one significant life lesson—be it in a Scripture, an anecdote you heard in a group meeting or a one-sentence chapter summary—that you will carry with you. Think of them as souvenirs from the journey!

Week Two

_____

_____

_____

Week Three

_____

_____

_____

Week Four

_____

_____

_____

Week Five

_____

_____

_____

Week Six

_____

_____

_____

Week Seven

_____

_____

_____

Week Eight

_____

_____

_____

Week Nine

_____

_____

_____

Week Ten

_____

_____

_____

Week Eleven

_____

_____

_____

Lord, thank You for all that You've taught me and all that You've accomplished in me and through me over the past weeks. Help me never to forget the things that You've spoken to my heart. Amen.

Day
7

REFLECTION AND APPLICATION

Father, please continue the good work that You've begun. Help me to be faithful to walk in the truth that You have shown me. Amen.

Now it's time for one last review of your original goals set in Week Two. At Week Six, you were able to assess your progress and/or adjust your goals as necessary. Since we're at the end of this study, determine whether or not you achieved each of your goals. If you did reach your goals, how will you maintain each of your achievements? If you didn't reach each goal, what must you start to do or continue to do to achieve success?

Emotional health

_____

_____

_____

_____

Spiritual health

_____

_____

_____

_____

Mental health

_____

_____

_____

_____

Physical health

_____

_____

_____

_____

Thank You, Lord, for bringing me all this way! Help me to finish strong and make the most of this new beginning! In Jesus' name, amen.

Notes

1. David Anderson, "Circling Upwards," email newsletter, March 3, 2010.
2. Lettie B. Cowman, *Streams in the Desert*, ed. James Reimann (Grand Rapids, MI: Zondervan, 2008), June 13.

Group Prayer Requests

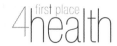

Today's Date: _____

Name	Request

Results

_____

_____

_____

_____

_____

_____

time to
celebrate!

To help shape your brief victory celebration testimony, work through the following questions in your prayer journal:

Day One: List some of the benefits you have gained by allowing the Lord to transform your life through this 12-week First Place 4 Health session. Be sure to list benefits you have received in the physical, mental, emotional and spiritual realms of your being.

Day Two: In what ways have you most significantly changed *mentally*? Have you seen a shift in the ways you think about yourself, food, your relationships or God? How has Scripture memory been a part of these shifts?

Day Three: In what ways have you most significantly changed *emotionally*? Have you begun to identify how your feelings influence your relationship to food and exercise? What are you doing to stay aware of your emotions, both positive and negative?

Day Four: In what ways have you most significantly changed *spiritually*? How has your relationship with God deepened? How has drawing closer to Him made a difference in the other three areas of your life?

Day Five: In what ways have you most significantly changed *physically*? Have you met or exceeded your weight/measurement goals? How has your health improved the past 12 weeks?

Day Six: Was there one person in your First Place 4 Health group who was particularly encouraging to you? How did their kindness make a difference in your First Place 4 Health journey?

Day Seven: Summarize the previous six questions into a one-page testimony, or "faith story," to share at your group's victory celebration.

May our gracious Lord bless and keep you as you continue to keep Him first in all things!

A New Beginning
leader discussion guide

For in-depth information, guidance and helpful tips about leading a successful First Place 4 Health group, study the *First Place 4 Health Leader's Guide*. In it, you will find valuable answers to most of your questions, as well as personal insights from many First Place 4 Health group leaders.

For the group meetings in this session, be sure to read and consider each week's discussion topics several days before the meeting—some questions and activities require supplies and/or planning to complete. Also, if you are leading a large group, plan to break into smaller groups for discussion and then come together as a large group to share your answers and responses. Make sure to appoint a capable leader for each small group so that discussions stay focused and on track (and be sure each group records their answers!).

week one: welcome to *a new beginning*

During this first week, welcome the members to your group, provide a brief overview of the First Place 4 Health program, explain what is expected of the participants at each of the weekly meetings, and collect the Member Surveys. (See the *First Place 4 Health Leader's Guide* for a detailed outline of how to conduct the first week's meeting.)

week two: making a fresh start

On Day One, participants were asked to describe how and when they first became "new creations" in Christ. Ask if anyone would like to briefly share their answer—their testimony.

Ask a volunteer to read 1 Corinthians 6:19-20. Have members discuss what this verse means when it says that our bodies are the "temple of the Holy Spirit" and that "we are not our own." Continue the discussion by asking how being overweight, unhealthy or out of balance hinders our relationships with God and others. Help the group understand that such a hindrance keeps us from living the life to which God has called us. Ask the group how living a balanced, healthy life honors God.

On a whiteboard or flip chart, list the seven characteristics the members studied from Day Four that, according to 2 Peter 1:5-8, we should exhibit to show we have faith.

On Day Five, participants were asked about the benefits of being obedient. Make sure the group members understand that according to Philippians 2:14-16, one of the benefits is that we "shine like stars in the universe"; we are examples—how we live, how we act, how we talk—of Christ for the unbelieving world to see. How we "shine" may influence whether an unbeliever comes to believe in Jesus.

Talk about setting goals. On a whiteboard or flip chart, make a list of keywords for goal setting. Explain that our goals should be *specific* and *measurable*. Otherwise, how will we know if we've achieved them? Goals should also be *reasonable*. Our expectations regarding weight loss, in particular, can tend to be a little unrealistic. Yes, we'll need to depend on God's grace and His strength to achieve any of our goals, but it should not take a miracle on the scale of the parting of the Red Sea!

With this in mind, invite group members to share one of their specific goals (emotional, spiritual, mental or physical) for the weeks ahead and one concrete step they plan to take toward achieving that goal.

As group members prepare to move forward into a new week, encourage them to let go of past failures and mistakes. Repeat the words of Winston Churchill on Day Six of this week's study: "Success is not final, failure is not fatal: it is the courage to continue that counts." Remind everyone that thanks to Jesus, we've all been given a new beginning, and we can all make a fresh start.

week three: learning from the past

Begin by inviting participants to share their successes—not just results from the scale—but any progress they've made, any positive steps they've taken toward their goals this past week.

On Day One, members were asked to read Deuteronomy 8:3-5 and identify four things that God's people needed to learn. As volunteers share their answers, list them on a whiteboard or a flip chart. (Answers should include humbleness, life is a gift from God, life is guaranteed to those who follow God's commands, and God disciplines His children.)

Discuss what giving Christ first place means. Ask what giving Christ first place looks like on a practical level in our daily lives.

Ephesians 4:32 tells us to "be kind and compassionate to one another." Discuss whether members have found that their own struggles have taught them to be more tolerant, more understanding and more compassionate when it comes to others' weaknesses.

Ask group members if they can identify reasons that past weight-loss efforts may have been unsuccessful. On a whiteboard or flip chart, write their answers. (Answers may include a lack of commitment, discipline or willpower; unrealistic expectations; unexpected obstacles; family crises or personal issues; an unbalanced diet or exercise routine that didn't prove liveable).

Discuss the important lessons that group members have learned from these experiences. Remind them that they will continue to get valuable feedback and learn important lessons—both from their failures and successes—as they participate in the First Place 4 Health program.

Bring in a piece of tapestry (or embroidery) that you can use as a visual example of the poem the group read on Day Six. (You might ask a volunteer to read the poem out loud.) Show the back of the tapestry, and point out that from one perspective, the tapestry may appear to be a mess—or at least an obscure, even random, arrangement of colors and threads. But turn it over and it becomes clear that there is, in fact, a carefully constructed pattern, a beautiful design.

Ask if anyone might be willing to give an example of something in his or her life that was difficult or painful, but from which God has brought good. Also ask if anyone has kept an object, a symbol or a record—a memorial—of what God has done for him or her. (In the context of a health and wellness program, it might be a piece of clothing that is now several sizes too big. Of course, it could also be something completely different, relevant to another aspect of a member's life.) If you have such an object, consider bringing it in to share with the group your own brief testimony.

Close by offering a prayer of thanksgiving for God's sovereignty, His wisdom, His patience and His love.

week four: living in the present

Welcome everyone to Week Four, and invite members to share any successes or victories from the previous week.

Discuss why it's important to live in the present—to be aware and alert and focused on choices before us today. Discuss what happens when we're distracted by living in the past or the future, what impact that can have on our emotions, and what impact our emotions have on our choices (see the introduction to the chapter).

On a whiteboard or flip chart, draw three columns with the headings: "Act Justly," "Love Mercy," "Walk Humbly." Go over in which category the Ten Commandments, the Shema, and the Golden Rule fit (see Day One). Ask members to volunteer other commandments from Scripture, and together decide under which broad category the commandment fits.

Ask participants to consider what it means to do what is right—to live a life of integrity—in the context of their First Place 4 Health journey. (Answers may include making healthy choices, being truthful and accurate in filling out their Live-It Tracker, keeping their commitment to exercise, and taking responsibility for poor choices rather than blaming other people or circumstances.)

The study on Day Four discussed how to be merciful and forgiving to those who have sinned against us. Note to the group that forgiveness does not mean pretending an offense didn't happen, that it didn't hurt or that it doesn't matter. It's not making excuses for others' sin against us or letting it continue without consequences. True forgiveness is choosing not to hold another's sin against them, because God doesn't hold our sin against us.

(Forgiveness can be a tough topic to handle in a brief weekly meeting—particularly when it isn't the focus of our study. For members who are really struggling with this issue, be prepared to privately recommend a Christian counselor, support group or some other resource your pastor or church may suggest.)

Have a volunteer read Matthew 11:28-30 and discuss what it means to be "yoked" to Jesus. Why does it require an attitude of humility on His part? Why does it require humility on our part? Also discuss how walking with God gives us rest.

Read the words of Hudson Taylor found in the reading for Day Seven: "A little thing is a little thing, but faithfulness in little things is a great thing." Discuss why this is true. Ask volunteers to share a little thing in which they have been faithful this week—any victory or success, no matter how small. Celebrate together!

Refer to Galatians 6:9 and challenge members to "not grow weary in doing good" this week but to keep moving forward—one day at a time, one step at a time, living in the present!

week five: leaning on Jesus

Welcome everyone and give them an opportunity to share any successes or victories they have experienced this past week.

Read 1 Corinthians 1:26-31. Ask members what encouragement they drew from this passage and the week's lesson overall. Have them turn to 1 Corinthians 10:13 and read it aloud together. Invite volunteers to share "a way out" that God provided for them this week or sometime in the past. For instance, did the phone ring right when they were reaching for an unhealthy food choice? Did a Scripture come to mind just as they were about to lose their patience with someone?

Have a volunteer (or three volunteers—one as the narrator, one as Jesus, and one as the tempter) read Matthew 4:1-11. Discuss the power of responding to temptation with Scripture. Ask if anyone has tried responding to temptation with his or her own logic or reasoning, and, if they did, what happened.

Ask volunteers to share which of the practical ways to lean on Jesus given on Day Six they found most helpful to them this week. On a whiteboard or flip chart, make a list of other tips that participants suggest.

Close with a prayer thanking God for using "cracked pots"—broken vessels—to reveal His glory, and for the great things He has done.

week six: looking ahead

Welcome everyone. Invite members to share any successes or victories from the previous week. Ask volunteers to share how the First Place 4 Health program has helped them focus on becoming more like Jesus.

Turn to 2 Peter 1:3-4. Discuss the implications of these verses. For example, if God has given us everything that we need, then is there any reason to doubt or fear? Is there any excuse for not doing what He's called us to? If we really believed these words, what impact would they have on our lives today?

Have someone read James 1:2-4 and James 1:12. Discuss what perseverance is and why it is so important. On a whiteboard or flip chart, make a list of the rewards (both for now and in eternity) for persevering in this journey of faith. Discuss what we can look forward to when we accomplish our goals.

Make sure that participants understand that they can experience peace when they give all of their concerns to God. Then discuss how God's peace can "guard" our hearts and minds (Philippians 4:7). (The *Amplified Bible* says it will "garrison and mount guard.")

Be prepared to help members who are struggling with their goals, who need to readjust their goals, or who need to set new ones. If they choose to share their struggles with the group, you can encourage a little brainstorming—others can share what type of goals they have set and what has worked for them. Otherwise, offer to speak with struggling members one on one after the group session. Ask questions and listen to their answers. Try to help them come up with ideas of their own. You can make a few suggestions, but resist the urge to tell them what they "must" or "should" do.

In closing, challenge members to stay focused on our ultimate goal of growing in our relationship with Jesus.

week seven: giving our best

Welcome everyone and invite members to share any successes or victories from the previous week.

Day One summarizes the theme and key points of the entire week's study. Have members take turns sharing their answers to each of the questions—from the perspective of their commitment to honor God through their participation in First Place 4 Health. For instance, what things would fall into the "whatever you do" category? Filling in your Live It Tracker, drinking your eight glasses of water, memorizing this week's verse.

Ask a volunteer to read Psalm 86:11-12. Invite participants to share the importance of having "an undivided" heart. Ask if anyone found a particular positive affirmation helpful to him or her this week, as he or she tried to break the habit of grumbling or complaining about "having" to be obedient.

On a whiteboard or flip chart, make a list of actions that the world might consider "radical" that are a reflection of our willingness to be obedient to God. (Answers may be specifically related to the First Place 4 Health journey or not. Answers also may include biblical examples, such as Joseph choosing forgiveness, Esther taking a stand, and the 12 disciples giving up everything to follow Jesus.)

Ask volunteers to tell which of the blessings of obedience speaks to them or motivates them the most. Review the parable of the talents retold on Day Six. Then read aloud the quote from Erma Bombeck. Invite members to share their reflections. Close by praying that the Holy Spirit would empower each group member to give God, for His glory, his or her best this week, in all that they do every day.

week eight: growing in grace

Welcome everyone and invite members to share any successes or victories from the previous week.

Introduce the subject of God's amazing grace. Ask volunteers to share what this grace means to them. Talk about the downward spiral mentioned on Day Two. Discuss how unresolved feelings of guilt over our mistakes and failures can lead to greater mistakes and failures, greater guilt and greater despair. Ask participants to explain what that looks like in terms of our First Place 4 Health journey. Discuss what we can do to escape from the spiral and turn the situation around.

Read the quote from Oswald Chambers on the power of obedience from Day Two. Next, have a volunteer read Titus 2:11-14. Ask volunteers to share one of the statements of faith that they created on Day Three: "By God's grace, I will . . ." Be prepared to share one of your own and to tell whether you repeated it to yourself in times of temptation or in other ways drew strength from it during the week.

Discuss the story of Jonah from Day Four and Day Five. Ahead of time, prepare a whiteboard or a piece of poster board with a simple outline of a large fish. Inside, print the prayer from Jonah 2:8-9. Recite it together. (If you have extra time to prepare this week, you can create mini versions of the poster—simple fish shapes cut from colored construction paper with the verses pasted on top for members to take home with them.)

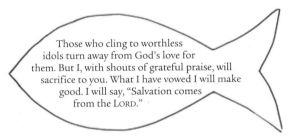

Those who cling to worthless idols turn away from God's love for them. But I, with shouts of grateful praise, will sacrifice to you. What I have vowed I will make good. I will say, "Salvation comes from the LORD."

Point out that two of the most important lessons the story of Jonah teaches us are (1) the miraculous, life-changing power of God's mercy and grace, and (2) the need to extend that grace to others.

week nine: surrendering to His lordship

Welcome everyone and invite members to share any successes or victories from the previous week.

On Day One, members were asked to consider what it means to call Jesus "Lord" and to identify to which of three groups they might belong. Discuss how all of this relates to our First Place 4 Health journey.

Emphasize that surrendering to the Lordship of Christ is an ongoing and continual process. Point out that surrendering to the Lordship of Jesus means that we're responsible to and accountable for our obedience to Him. In light of this, invite members to share with their prayer partners an area in which they are struggling to be obedient, and have them ask their partners to call or email them to check on their progress and hold them accountable this week.

Invite volunteers to share stories of experiences through which they have learned "the joy of self-sacrifice" that Oswald Chambers talked about. (Stories may or may not be specifically related to their First Place 4 Health journey.)

Ask a volunteer to read Jeremiah 18:1-6. Discuss the encouragement found in the last paragraph on Day Six. If you have access to any clay or pottery that might serve as a good visual aid, bring it with you. You could also (or instead) purchase a small inexpensive tub of play dough (the kind that is used in treat bags or as party favors) for each member. Print Isaiah 64:8 on strips of paper and tape one over each label.

week ten: standing by faith

Before you begin, on a flip chart or piece of poster board, draw a simple outline of an open, outstretched hand; or mount a large picture of a hand you've found online. As you welcome and greet group members this week, direct them to the outline or picture, and ask them to write their names on the palm of the hand, just as God says He has engraved their names on His palms (see Isaiah 49).

Discuss some of the "giants" that people face when they try to make significant life changes. Many people get so discouraged just thinking about these giants that they never try. Ask volunteers to share examples of how God has been training them for battle—teaching them a skill or strategy to use on their First Place 4 Health journey. Consider listing these on a whiteboard or flip chart.

Talk about the prayer of Jehoshaphat from Day Six. Discuss why it had such power, and why praise and worship so often play such an important role in defeating the enemy of our souls. Ask for opinions about the king's battle strategy.

With two weeks left to go in this study, ask how members can use what they've learned this week to help them stand strong and stay strong, all the way to the finish. Close by reading 1 Thessalonians 5:23-24 as a benediction.

week eleven: soaring in the strength of the Spirit

Welcome everyone and invite members to share any successes or victories from the previous week.

Have a volunteer read Isaiah 40:28-30 aloud, and then review Pastor Dave's story about the eagles from the introduction to the chapter. Ask what insights members gained from this story—or others they have heard. (Eagles have many characteristics that lend themselves to spiritual comparisons or allegories, and there are a lot of sermons preached on what it means to soar like an eagle!)

Talk about what it means to hope in the Lord, to wait on the Lord, and to trust in the Lord. Discuss what these mean in the context of our First Place 4 Health journey—how we hope in the Lord, wait on Him or trust in Him as we're working to make healthy lifestyle changes.

On Day Two, participants learned that we are to walk in obedience to God's Word while we wait on Him. Discuss what this looks like for First Place 4 Health members. In other words, what part of this journey is God's part—His responsibility, the things that only He can do—and what is our responsibility, or our part?

On Day Four, members were asked to consider what things might be hindering them or holding them back. Their answers may be very personal, but ask volunteers to share or perhaps give a general example of the kinds of obstacles that can be handled alone and the obstacles with which we need help. Ask for ideas and suggestions about how specifically to address each obstacle.

Remind everyone of the words of Zechariah 4:6. Ultimately, it's not by our might or by our power (human strength, determination or willpower) but by God's Spirit that the victory is won!

Prepare ahead of time a small suitcase filled with a few of your souvenirs from your First Place 4 Health journey. You might include the tapestry from Week Three, a cracked pot to represent Week Five, a fish from Week Eight, and some clay or play dough from Week Nine—as well as some of your own personal items. Share a little of what God has been teaching you the past 11 weeks as you review the key themes (use the table of contents as an outline of what's been covered). Let members know that next week there will be an opportunity for each of them to share their own testimony.

Close with a prayer asking God to be with each member during this last week and help them to finish this session—this part of their lifelong journey—strong!

week twelve: time to celebrate!

Even though most of your meeting this week will be a victory celebration, take some time at the beginning of the meeting to talk about how much God loves each person in the group and how each of us is called to love our brothers and sisters in Christ. (See "Planning a Victory Celebration" in the *First Place 4 Health Leader's Guide* for ideas about throwing a successful celebration for your group.)

For the rest of the study time, allow each member to tell his or her *A New Beginning* story. Give members an equal opportunity to share the goals they set for themselves at the beginning of the session and talk about the challenges and good things God has done for them throughout the process. Don't allow the more talkative group members to monopolize all the time. Even the quiet members need an opportunity to share their stories and successes! Even those who have not met their goals have still been part of the journey, so allow them to share and talk about why they did not succeed.

Making a commitment to continue in First Place 4 Health is an important part of victory. Be sure to talk about your group's future plans, and make each person feel welcome to continue to journey with you.

End your victory celebration by reading aloud this prayer based on 2 Peter 3:18:

Lord, we thank You for this new beginning You have given each one of us. And we thank You that You always finish what You start. Help us all to persevere on the path You've shown us, to continue to "grow in the grace and knowledge of our Lord and Savior Jesus Christ. To Him be glory both now and forever! Amen."

First Place 4 Health menu plans

Each menu plan is based on approximately 1,400 to 1,500 calories per day. All recipe and menu exchanges were determined using the Master-Cook software, a program that accesses a database containing more than 6,000 food items prepared using the United States Department of Agriculture (USDA) publications and information from food manufacturers. As with any nutritional program, MasterCook calculates the nutritional values of the recipes based on ingredients. Nutrition may vary due to how the food is prepared, where the food comes from, soil content, season, ripeness, processing and method of preparation. For these reasons, please use the recipes and menu plans as approximate guides. Consult a physician and/or a registered dietitian before starting a weight-loss program.

For those who need more calories, add the following to the 1,400-calorie plan:

- 1,800 calories: 2 ounce equivalent of meat, 3 ounce equivalent of bread, ½ cup vegetable serving, 1 tsp. fat

- 2,000 calories: 2 ounce equivalent of meat, 4 ounce equivalent of bread, ½ cup vegetable serving, 3 tsp. fat

- 2,200 calories: 2 ounce equivalent of meat, 5 ounce equivalent of bread, ½ cup vegetable serving, ½ cup fruit serving, 5 tsp. fat

- 2,400 calories: 2 ounce equivalent of meat, 6 ounce equivalent of bread, 1 cup vegetable serving, ½ cup fruit serving, 6 tsp. fat

First Week Grocery List

Produce
- [ ] apples
- [ ] apricots, dried
- [ ] basil
- [ ] berries
- [ ] capers
- [ ] carrots
- [ ] celery
- [ ] cilantro
- [ ] cremini mushrooms
- [ ] currants
- [ ] garlic, cloves
- [ ] garlic, minced
- [ ] green bell pepper
- [ ] green onions
- [ ] leeks
- [ ] lemons
- [ ] mint leaves
- [ ] parsley
- [ ] parsnips
- [ ] peaches
- [ ] pineapple
- [ ] raisins, golden
- [ ] red onion
- [ ] romaine lettuce
- [ ] shallots
- [ ] spinach leaves, baby
- [ ] spring mix salad greens
- [ ] tomato
- [ ] yellow onion
- [ ] zucchini

Baking/Cooking Products
- [ ] baking powder
- [ ] baking soda
- [ ] canola oil
- [ ] chocolate, semisweet
- [ ] flour, all-purpose
- [ ] flour, whole-wheat
- [ ] nonstick cooking spray
- [ ] olive oil, extra virgin
- [ ] sugar
- [ ] turbinado sugar
- [ ] vanilla extract

Spices
- [ ] allspice, ground
- [ ] black pepper
- [ ] cayenne pepper
- [ ] chili powder
- [ ] cinnamon, ground
- [ ] cumin, ground
- [ ] curry powder
- [ ] fajita seasoning mix
- [ ] oregano, dried
- [ ] salt

Nuts/Seeds
- [ ] almonds
- [ ] flaxseeds, golden
- [ ] sesame seeds
- [ ] sunflower seeds
- [ ] walnuts

Condiments, Spreads and Sauces
- [ ] almond butter
- [ ] barbecue sauce
- [ ] dressing, light Ranch
- [ ] honey
- [ ] hot pepper sauce (such as Frank's RedHot®)

- ❑ mayonnaise, reduced-fat
- ❑ salsa
- ❑ white wine vinegar

Breads, Cereals and Pasta

- ❑ bran flakes
- ❑ bread, whole-grain
- ❑ breadcrumbs, dry
- ❑ breadsticks
- ❑ chips, baked
- ❑ dinner rolls, whole-grain
- ❑ English muffin, whole-wheat
- ❑ lasagna noodles
- ❑ linguine
- ❑ oats, rolled
- ❑ rye bread
- ❑ saltine crackers
- ❑ sandwich bun, whole-wheat
- ❑ spaghetti
- ❑ tortillas, corn
- ❑ tortillas, flour
- ❑ tortillas, whole-wheat
- ❑ wheat germ
- ❑ whole-grain puffed cereal

Canned Foods

- ❑ black beans, low-sodium
- ❑ chicken broth, low-sodium
- ❑ corn kernels
- ❑ fruit cups
- ❑ garbanzo beans
- ❑ tomato paste
- ❑ tomatoes, diced and undrained
- ❑ vegetable broth

Dairy Products

- ❑ bleu cheese, crumbled
- ❑ butter

- ❑ buttermilk, nonfat
- ❑ cheese, cheddar
- ❑ cheese, Monterey Jack, with jalapeño peppers
- ❑ cheese, Parmigiano-Reggiano
- ❑ cheese, Provolone, reduced-fat
- ❑ cottage cheese, low-fat
- ❑ Mexican cheese blend, reduced-fat, shredded
- ❑ sour cream, reduced-fat
- ❑ yogurt, light lemon or vanilla
- ❑ yogurt, plain

Juices

- ❑ orange juice
- ❑ lemon juice
- ❑ lime juice

Frozen Foods

- ❑ Lean Cuisine Grilled Chicken Caesar Pasta Bowl®
- ❑ stir-fry bell peppers and onions (1 bag)

Meat and Poultry

- ❑ chicken
- ❑ chicken breast halves, boneless, skinless
- ❑ chicken breast, rotisserie
- ❑ chicken tenders
- ❑ eggs
- ❑ egg beaters
- ❑ salmon, smoked
- ❑ sirloin, ground
- ❑ turkey breast
- ❑ turkey, ground and lean
- ❑ turkey sausage links, hot Italian

First Week Meals and Recipes

DAY 1

Breakfast

Cereal Sundae

¾ cup bran flakes   2 tbsp. walnuts
6 oz. light lemon or vanilla yogurt

Top yogurt with bran flakes and walnuts. Serves 1.

Nutritional Information: 298 calories; 10g fat (28% calories from fat); 15g protein; 45g carbohydrate; 8g dietary fiber; 2mg cholesterol; 358mg sodium.

Lunch

Lean Cuisine Pasta Bowl

1 (12-oz.) Lean Cuisine Grilled   1 cup carrot sticks
  Chicken Caesar Pasta Bowl®   ½ cup light Ranch dressing

Nutritional Information: 392 calories; 11g fat (24% calories from fat); 15g protein; 62g carbohydrate; 8g dietary fiber; 9mg cholesterol; 1,208mg sodium.

Dinner

Mushroom and Provolone Patty Melts

1 lb. ground sirloin   1½ tsp. all-purpose flour
1 tbsp. olive oil   ¼ cup water
¼ cup thinly sliced yellow onion   8 (1.1-oz.) slices rye bread
⅛ tsp. salt   4 (¾-oz.) slices reduced-fat provolone
⅛ tsp. black pepper   cheese
1 (8-oz.) package sliced cremini   nonstick cooking spray
  mushrooms

Heat a large nonstick skillet over medium-high heat. Shape beef into 4 (4-inch) patties. Coat pan with nonstick cooking spray and add patties. Cook patties 4 minutes on each side or until done. Next, heat oil in a separate medium-sized skillet over medium-high heat. Add onion, salt, pepper and mushrooms and sauté for 3 minutes. Sprinkle flour over the mushroom mixture and cook 1 minute, stirring constantly. Stir in water and cook for 30 seconds or until thick. Remove from heat and keep warm. When the patties are done, remove them from the large skillet. Wipe the pan clean and heat over medium-high heat. Coat one side of each bread slice with nonstick cooking spray. Place 4 bread slices, coated sides down, in pan. Top each with 1 patty, 1 cheese slice, and one-fourth of the mushroom mixture. Top with the remaining bread slices and coat with nonstick cooking spray. Cook for 2 minutes on each side or until browned. Serve with mixed fruit salad and baked chips. Serves 4.

Nutritional Information: 416 calories; 17g fat (28% calories from fat); 30g protein; 34g carbohydrate; 4g dietary fiber; 42mg cholesterol; 708mg sodium.

DAY 2

Breakfast

Breakfast Taco

2 corn tortillas
2 tbsp. shredded reduced-fat
   cheddar cheese

½ cup liquid egg substitute (such
   as Egg Beaters®)
1 tbsp. salsa

Scramble egg substitute. Fill each corn tortilla with ½ cup of egg substitute and 1 tablespoon cheese and salsa. Serve with 1 cup orange juice. Serves 1.

Nutritional Information: 245 calories; 6g fat (24% calories from fat); 22g protein; 25g carbohydrate; 3g dietary fiber; 4mg cholesterol; 459mg sodium.

Lunch

Fajita Lasagna

1 lb. extra lean ground beef
3 cups salsa
1 (1.4-oz.) packet fajita seasoning mix
12 lasagna noodles
nonstick cooking spray

1 (16-oz.) bag of frozen stir-fry bell
   peppers and onions, thawed and
   drained
2½ cups reduced-fat shredded Mexican cheese blend

Heat oven to 350° F. Coat the bottom and sides of a 13″ x 9″ x 2″ baking dish with nonstick cooking spray and set aside. Brown the ground beef in a nonstick skillet over medium heat, stirring occasionally, and then drain and stir in salsa and seasoning mix. Heat to boiling, stirring constantly. Layer in a baking dish in the following order: ½ cup meat sauce, spread over bottom of pan; 4 lasagna noodles, laid lengthwise on top of meat sauce; 1½ cups meat sauce, spread over the noodles; ½ bag stir-fry veggie mixture, spread over meat sauce; 1 cup cheese, sprinkled over stir-fry vegetables. Repeat in the same order and top with the remaining 4 noodles. Cover the noodles completely with the remaining sauce. Bake for 25 to 30 minutes and then top with the remaining cheese. Let stand for 12 minutes before cutting. Serve each with 1 apple and 1 cup spinach salad with 2 tablespoons light dressing. Serves 8.

Nutritional Information: 293 calories; 15g fat (46% calories from fat); 21g protein; 18g carbohydrate; 2g dietary fiber; 50mg cholesterol; 1,078mg sodium.

....

Dinner

Spaghetti with Sausage and Tomato Sauce

8 oz. hot Italian turkey sausage links
8 oz. uncooked spaghetti
1 (28-oz.) can no-salt-added whole tomatoes, undrained
2 tbsp. olive oil
½ tsp. crushed red pepper
5 garlic cloves, minced
1 tsp. sugar
½ tsp. salt
¼ cup torn fresh basil
½ (2 oz.) cup shaved Parmigiano-Reggiano cheese

Preheat the broiler. Arrange the sausage on a small baking sheet and broil the sausages for 5 minutes on each side or until done. Remove the pan from the oven (do not turn the broiler off). Cut sausage into ¼-inch-thick slices and arrange the slices in a single layer on the baking sheet. Broil the sausage slices for 2 minutes or until browned. Next, cook the pasta according to package directions, omitting salt and fat, and drain. Place the tomatoes in a food processor and process until almost smooth. Heat the olive oil in a large nonstick skillet over medium-high heat. Add crushed red pepper and minced garlic and sauté for 1 minute. Stir in tomatoes, sugar and salt and cook for 4 minutes or until slightly thick. Add sausage and cooked pasta to pan and toss well. Top with fresh basil and Parmigiano-Reggiano. Serve with mixed green salad with light dressing and whole-grain dinner roll. Serves 4.

Nutritional Information: 460 calories; 17g fat (33% calories from fat); 24g protein; 53.3g carbohydrate; 4g dietary fiber; 57mg cholesterol; 895mg sodium.

DAY 3

Breakfast

Healthy Whole-grain Waffles

1 cup whole-wheat flour
1 cup all-purpose flour
1½ tsp. baking powder
½ tsp. salt
¼ tsp. baking soda
2 cups nonfat buttermilk

1 large egg, separated
1 tbsp. canola oil
1 tbps. vanilla extract (optional)
2 large egg whites
2 tbsp. sugar

Stir the whole-wheat flour, all-purpose flour, baking powder, salt and baking soda in a large bowl. Whisk the buttermilk, egg yolk, oil and vanilla (optional) in a separate bowl. Add the wet ingredients to the dry ingredients and stir with a wooden spoon until just moistened. Beat the 3 egg whites in a grease-free mixing bowl with an electric mixer until soft peaks form. Add sugar and continue beating the egg whites until they are stiff and glossy. Whisk one-quarter of the beaten egg whites into the batter and then fold in the remaining beaten egg whites with a rubber spatula. Preheat a waffle iron. Brush the surface lightly with oil and fill the waffle iron two-thirds full of batter. Cook until the waffles are crisp and golden (about 5 to 6 minutes). Repeat with the remaining batter, brushing the surface with oil before cooking each batch. Serve with mixed fruit cup and 1 cup skim milk. Serves 8.

Nutritional Information: 241 calories; 4g fat (15% calories from fat); 11g protein; 41g carbohydrate; 3g dietary fiber; 37mg cholesterol; 450mg sodium.

Lunch

Barbecue Chicken Sandwich

(**Note:** This is a great way to use leftover chicken!)
½ cup shredded cooked chicken
¼ cup shredded carrots
2 tbsp. barbecue sauce

2 tsp. light Ranch dressing
1 small whole-wheat sandwich bun
1 leaf romaine lettuce

Combine chicken, carrots and barbecue sauce in a bowl. Spread Ranch dressing on the bun and top with the chicken mixture and lettuce. Serve with baked chips. Serves 1.

Nutritional Information: 323 calories; 8g fat (23% calories from fat); 26g protein; 37g carbohydrates; 4g dietary fiber; 62mg cholesterol; 729mg sodium.

Dinner

Chicken with Lemon-leek Linguine

6 oz. uncooked linguine	3 garlic cloves, thinly sliced
4 (6-oz.) skinless, boneless chicken breast halves	1½ cups leeks, trimmed, cut in half lengthwise and thinly sliced
½ tsp. salt, divided	½ cup fat-free, lower-sodium chicken broth
¼ tsp. black pepper	
¼ cup all-purpose flour	2 tbsp. lemon juice
3 tbsp. butter, divided	2 tbsp. chopped fresh flat-leaf parsley

Cook pasta according to package directions, omitting salt and fat. Drain and keep warm. Place the chicken between 2 sheets of heavy-duty plastic wrap and pound to an even thickness using a meat mallet or small heavy skillet. Sprinkle the chicken with ¼ teaspoon salt and pepper. Place flour in a shallow dish and dredge the chicken in the flour, shaking to remove excess. Next, heat 1 tablespoon butter in a large nonstick skillet over medium-high heat. Add chicken and cook for 3 minutes on each side or until done. Remove the chicken from pan and keep warm. Melt 1 tablespoon butter in a skillet over medium-high heat. Add garlic, leeks and ¼ tsp. salt and sauté for 4 minutes. Add the broth and juice and cook for 2 minutes or until liquid is reduced by half. Remove from the heat and stir in 1 tablespoon butter. Add the pasta to the leek mixture and toss well to combine. Serve the chicken over the pasta mixture and sprinkle with parsley. Serves 4.

Nutritional Information: 474 calories; 12g fat (22% calories from fat); 46.8g protein; 44g carbohydrate; 2.3g dietary fiber; 121mg cholesterol; 592mg sodium.

DAY 4

Breakfast

Egg and Salmon Sandwich

½ tsp. extra-virgin olive oil	½ tsp. capers, rinsed and chopped (optional)
1 tbsp. finely chopped red onion	
2 large egg whites, beaten	1 slice tomato
salt, pinch	1 whole-wheat English muffin, split and toasted
1 oz. smoked salmon	

Heat oil in a small nonstick skillet over medium heat. Add onion and cook, stirring, until it begins to soften (about 1 minute). Add the egg whites, salt and capers (optional) and cook, stirring constantly, until the whites are set (about 30 seconds). To make the sandwich, layer the egg whites, smoked salmon and tomato on an English muffin. Serve with 1 cup orange juice. Serves 1.

Nutritional Information: 214 calories; 5g fat (21% calories from fat); 19g protein; 25g carbohydrate; 3g dietary fiber; 7mg cholesterol; 670mg sodium.

Lunch

Vegetable Bean Soup

1 tbsp. olive oil
1 medium onion, chopped
2 cloves garlic, crushed with press
1½ tsp. curry powder
1½ tsp. ground cumin
¼ tsp. salt
1 cup water
1 (14½-oz.) can diced tomatoes
1 (14- to 15-oz.) can reduced-sodium chicken broth or vegetable broth

1 (15- to 19-oz.) can garbanzo beans (chickpeas), rinsed and drained
12 oz. carrots, peeled and cut into 1-inch chunks
12 oz. parsnips, peeled and cut into 1-inch chunks
1 large zucchini, cut into ½-inch chunks
¼ cup loosely packed fresh mint leaves, chopped

Heat oil in a 5- to 6-quart saucepot on medium until hot. Add onion and cook 8 to 10 minutes or until tender, stirring occasionally. Stir in garlic, curry, cumin and ¼ teaspoon salt. Cook for 30 seconds, stirring constantly. Add tomatoes, broth, beans, carrots, parsnips and water and heat to boiling on medium-high. Reduce the heat to medium and cover and cook for 10 minutes. Stir in the zucchini and cover and cook for 10 to 15 minutes longer or until vegetables are tender. Remove the saucepot from the heat and stir in mint. Serve with 6 saltine crackers. Serves 4.

Nutritional Information: 335 calories; 6g fat (17% calories from fat); 12g protein; 62g carbohydrate; 15g dietary fiber; 0mg cholesterol; 1,030mg sodium.

Dinner

Chicken Milanese with Spring Greens

¾ tsp. fresh lemon juice
¾ tsp. white wine vinegar
½ tsp. minced shallots
¼ tsp. salt, divided

sugar, dash
2 (6-oz.) skinless, boneless chicken breasts
⅓ cup breadcrumbs, dry

2 tbsp. grated Parmigiano-Reggiano
cheese
2 tbsp. all-purpose flour
1 egg white, lightly beaten
¼ tsp. black pepper, divided

5 tsp. olive oil, divided
2 cups packed spring mix salad
greens
2 lemon wedges

Combine lemon juice, vinegar, shallots, ⅛ teaspoon salt and sugar and let stand for 15 minutes. Place the chicken between 2 sheets of heavy-duty plastic wrap and pound to ½-inch thickness using a meat mallet or small heavy skillet. Combine breadcrumbs and cheese in a shallow dish; place the flour in a separate shallow dish; and place the egg white in a third shallow dish. Sprinkle chicken with ⅛ teaspoon salt and ⅛ teaspoon pepper. Dredge the chicken in the flour, then dip in the egg white, and then dredge in the breadcrumb mixture. Place the chicken on a wire rack and let stand for 5 minutes. Next, heat 1 tablespoon oil in a large nonstick skillet over medium-high heat. Add the chicken and cook for 3 minutes. Turn the chicken over and cook for 2 minutes or until browned and done. Add 2 teaspoons oil and ⅛ teaspoon pepper to the shallot mixture and stir with a whisk. Add in the greens and toss gently. Place the chicken breast half on each of 2 plates and serve with lemon wedges. Also serve with 1 cup mixed green salad with light dressing and one breadstick. Serves 2.

Nutritional Information: 402 calories; 15g (35% calories from fat); 46g protein; 187g carbohydrate; 1.4g dietary fiber; 102mg cholesterol; 539mg sodium.

DAY 5

Breakfast

Berry Breakfast Smoothie
1¼ cups fresh berries
¾ cup low-fat plain yogurt
½ cup orange juice
2 tbsp. nonfat dry milk

1 tbsp. toasted wheat germ
1 tbsp. honey
½ tsp. vanilla extract

Place berries, yogurt, orange juice, dry milk, wheat germ, honey and vanilla in a blender and blend until smooth. Serves 1.

Nutritional Information: 432 calories; 3g fat (7% calories from fat); 20g protein; 77g carbohydrate; 7g dietary fiber; 15mg cholesterol; 250mg sodium.

Lunch

Tortilla Pie

1 cup frozen corn kernels
2 green onions, thinly sliced
1 tsp. ground cumin
1½ cups salsa
1 (15- to 19-oz.) can low-sodium
  black beans, rinsed and drained

4 burrito-size flour tortillas
  (96% fat-free)
1 (8-oz.) package reduced-fat shredded Mexican cheese blend
2 tbsp. chopped fresh cilantro leaves
nonstick cooking spray

Preheat oven to 450° F. Spray a large cookie sheet with nonstick cooking spray. Spray a 12-inch nonstick skillet with nonstick cooking spray and place over medium heat. Add frozen corn, green onions and cumin and cook for 3 minutes or until the corn thaws. Remove the skillet from the heat and stir in salsa and beans. Place 1 tortilla on cookie sheet and top with 1 cup of the bean mixture and ½ cup cheese. Repeat, starting with the tortilla, to make 2 more layers. Top with the remaining tortilla and cheese. Bake the pie for 10 minutes or until heated through. Carefully transfer the pie to a cutting board and sprinkle with chopped cilantro. With sharp knife, cut into wedges to serve. Serves 4.

Nutritional Information: 440 calories; 13g fat (27% calories from fat); 26g protein; 58g carbohydrate; 21g dietary fiber; 41mg cholesterol; 420mg sodium.

Dinner

Pepper Jack, Chicken and Peach Quesadillas

1 tsp. honey
½ tsp. lime juice
½ cup reduced-fat sour cream
4 (8-inch) flour tortillas
¾ cup shredded Monterey Jack
  cheese with jalapeño peppers

1 cup chopped skinless, boneless
  rotisserie chicken breast
1 cup thinly sliced, peeled firm ripe
  peaches
4 tsp. chopped fresh cilantro
nonstick cooking spray

Combine honey and lime juice in a small bowl, stirring well with a whisk. Stir sour cream into the honey mixture and cover and chill until ready to serve. Place tortillas flat on a work surface. Sprinkle 3 tablespoons of the cheese over half of each tortilla, and then top each tortilla with ¼ cup chicken, ¼ cup peaches and 1 teaspoon cilantro. Fold tortillas in half. Heat a large nonstick skillet over medium-high heat. Coat pan with nonstick cooking spray, place 2 quesadillas in the pan, and top quesadillas with a cast-iron or other heavy skillet. Cook 1½ minutes on each side or until the tortillas are crisp and lightly browned (leave the cast-iron skillet on the quesadillas as they cook). Remove the quesadillas from pan, set aside and keep warm. Repeat this procedure with the remaining quesadillas. Cut each quesadilla into wedges and serve with sauce. Serves 4.

Nutritional Information: 364 calories; 16g fat (40% calories from fat); 21g protein; 34g carbohydrate; 2g dietary fiber; 68mg cholesterol; 485mg sodium.

DAY 6

....

Breakfast
Almond Honey Power Bar

1 cup old-fashioned rolled oats
¼ cup slivered almonds
¼ cup sunflower seeds
1 tbsp. flaxseeds, preferably golden
1 tbsp. sesame seeds
1 cup unsweetened whole-grain
   puffed cereal
⅓ cup currants

⅓ cup chopped dried apricots
⅓ cup chopped golden raisins
¼ cup creamy almond butter
¼ cup turbinado sugar
¼ cup honey
½ tsp. vanilla extract
⅛ tsp. salt
nonstick cooking spray

Preheat oven to 350° F. Coat an 8″ square pan with cooking spray. Spread oats, almonds, sunflower seeds, flaxseeds and sesame seeds on a large, rimmed baking sheet. Bake until the oats are lightly toasted and the nuts are fragrant, shaking the pan halfway through (about 10 minutes). Transfer the mixture to a large bowl. Add cereal, currants, apricots and raisins and toss to combine. Combine almond butter, sugar, honey, vanilla and salt in a small saucepan. Cook over medium-low heat, stirring frequently, until the mixture bubbles lightly (about 2 to 5 minutes). Immediately pour the almond butter mixture over the dry ingredients and mix with a spoon or spatula until no dry spots remain. Transfer to the prepared pan. Lightly coat your hands with the nonstick cooking spray and press the mixture down firmly to make an even layer (wait until the mixture cools slightly, if necessary). Refrigerate until firm (about 30 minutes) and cut into 8 bars. (Note: You can store the power bars in an airtight container at room temperature or in the refrigerator for up to one week, or in the freezer for up to one month). Serves 8.

Nutritional Information: 244 calories; 10g fat (37% calories from fat); 5g protein; 38g carbohydrate; 3g dietary fiber; 0mg cholesterol; 74mg sodium.

....

Lunch

Buffalo Chicken Wrap

2 tbsp. hot pepper sauce (such as Frank's RedHot®)
3 tbsp. white vinegar, divided
¼ tsp. cayenne pepper
2 tsp. extra-virgin olive oil
1 lb. chicken tenders
2 tbsp. reduced-fat mayonnaise

2 tbsp. nonfat plain yogurt
ground pepper, to taste
¼ cup crumbled bleu cheese
4 (8-inch) whole-wheat tortillas
1 cup shredded romaine lettuce
1 cup sliced celery
1 large tomato, diced

Whisk hot pepper sauce, 2 tablespoons vinegar and cayenne pepper in a medium bowl. Heat oil in a large nonstick skillet over medium-high heat. Add chicken tenders and cook until cooked through and no longer pink in the middle (about 3 to 4 minutes per side). Add the chicken tenders to the bowl with the hot pepper sauce and toss to coat well. Whisk mayonnaise, yogurt, pepper and the remaining 1 tablespoon vinegar in a small bowl. Stir in the bleu cheese. To assemble the wraps, first lay a tortilla on a work surface or plate. Spread with 1 tablespoon bleu cheese sauce and top with one-fourth of the chicken, lettuce, celery and tomato. Drizzle with some of the hot sauce remaining in the bowl and roll into a wrap sandwich. Repeat with the remaining tortillas. Serves 4.

Nutritional Information: 275 calories; 8g fat (26% calories from fat); 24g protein; 29g carbohydrate; 3g dietary fiber; 55 mg cholesterol; 756 mg sodium.

....

Dinner

Cincinnati Turkey Chili

4 oz. uncooked spaghetti
8 oz. lean ground turkey
1½ cups pre-chopped onion, divided

1 cup chopped green bell pepper
1 tbsp. bottled minced garlic
1 tbsp. chili powder

2 tbsp. tomato paste
1 tsp. ground cumin
1 tsp. dried oregano
¼ tsp. ground cinnamon
⅛ tsp. ground allspice
½ cup fat-free, less-sodium chicken broth
1 (15-oz.) can kidney beans, rinsed and drained

1 (14½-oz.) can diced tomatoes, undrained
2½ tbsp. chopped semisweet chocolate
¼ tsp. salt
¾ cup shredded sharp cheddar cheese
nonstick cooking spray

Cook pasta according to package directions, omitting salt and fat. Drain and set aside. Heat a Dutch oven (or any large heavy pot with lid) over medium-high heat. Coat pan with nonstick cooking spray and add turkey. Cook for 3 minutes, stirring to crumble. Add 1 cup onion, bell pepper and garlic and sauté for 3 minutes. Stir in the chili powder, tomato paste, cumin, oregano, cinnamon and allspice and cook for 1 minute. Add broth, beans and tomatoes and bring to a boil. Cover, reduce heat and simmer for 20 minutes, stirring occasionally. Remove from heat and stir in chocolate and salt. Serve the chili over spaghetti and top with the remaining ½ cup onion and cheese. Serve with 6 saltine crackers. Serves 4.

Nutritional Information: 408 calories; 14g fat (31% calories from fat); 24g protein; 47g carbohydrate; 8g dietary fiber; 67mg cholesterol; 765mg sodium.

DAY 7

Breakfast

Breakfast Parfait

¾ cup low-fat cottage cheese, or low-fat plain yogurt
2 tsp. toasted wheat germ

1 cup pineapple chunks (can use papaya chunks or cling peaches)

Place cottage cheese (or yogurt) in a small bowl. Top with fruit and sprinkle with wheat germ. Serves 1.

Nutritional Information: 248 calories; 2g fat (8% calories from fat); 23g protein; 35g carbohydrate; 3g dietary fiber; 7mg cholesterol; 24mg sodium.

Lunch

Garden Turkey Sandwich with Lemon Mayo

1 tsp. grated lemon peel
1 tbsp. low-fat mayonnaise
2 slices whole-grain bread
2 oz. turkey breast, sliced

1 small tomato, sliced
1 cup loosely packed baby spinach
 leaves

Stir the grated lemon peel into the mayonnaise and spread on both slices of bread. On one slice of the bread, alternately layer spinach leaves, turkey and tomato, starting and ending with spinach. Top with the second bread slice. Serves 1.

Nutritional Information: 300 calories; 7g fat (21% calories from fat); 26g protein; 33g carbohydrate; 13g dietary fiber; 57mg cholesterol; 320mg sodium.

Dinner

Small Caesar or house salad with
 light dressing on the side
1 cup steamed vegetables

Split entrée of chicken piccata or
 chicken marsala
1½ cups pasta with marinara sauce

Order the above items at an Italian restaurant of your choice. Serves 1.

Nutritional Information: 632 calories; 29g fat (42% calories from fat); 21g protein; 68g carbohydrate; 9g dietary fiber; 30mg cholesterol; 1,663mg sodium.

Second Week Grocery List

Produce
- ❑ apple
- ❑ avocados
- ❑ berries
- ❑ Boston lettuce
- ❑ broccoli
- ❑ carrots
- ❑ celery
- ❑ chives
- ❑ cilantro
- ❑ eggplants
- ❑ fresh fruit salad
- ❑ garlic, minced
- ❑ grape tomatoes
- ❑ green onion
- ❑ lemon
- ❑ lettuce
- ❑ lime
- ❑ orange
- ❑ pears
- ❑ plum tomatoes
- ❑ red onions
- ❑ romaine lettuce
- ❑ snow peas
- ❑ spinach, baby
- ❑ tomatoes
- ❑ zucchini

Baking/Cooking Products
- ❑ canola oil
- ❑ extra virgin olive oil
- ❑ flour, all-purpose
- ❑ honey
- ❑ maple syrup
- ❑ nonstick cooking spray
- ❑ olive oil
- ❑ sesame oil, dark
- ❑ vanilla extract

Spices
- ❑ basil
- ❑ black pepper, ground
- ❑ cinnamon
- ❑ nutmeg
- ❑ oregano
- ❑ paprika
- ❑ pumpkin pie spice
- ❑ red pepper, ground
- ❑ salt
- ❑ thyme

Nuts/Seeds
- ❑ almonds
- ❑ hazelnuts
- ❑ pecans

Condiments, Spreads and Sauces
- ❑ Dijon mustard
- ❑ horseradish
- ❑ hot chili sauce
- ❑ mayonnaise, canola
- ❑ mayonnaise, fat-free
- ❑ mustard
- ❑ pasta sauce
- ❑ Ranch dressing, light
- ❑ salsa
- ❑ soy sauce, low-sodium

Breads, Cereals and Pasta
- ❑ bagels, whole-grain
- ❑ baked tortilla chips

- ❑ basmati rice
- ❑ bread, peasant
- ❑ bread, whole-wheat
- ❑ breadsticks
- ❑ corn flake cereal, whole-grain
- ❑ couscous
- ❑ dinner roll, whole-grain
- ❑ flour tortillas, reduced-fat
- ❑ French bread baguette
- ❑ granola bar, whole-grain crunchy
- ❑ oatmeal, plain instant
- ❑ Panko (Japanese breadcrumbs), whole-wheat

Canned Foods
- ❑ black beans
- ❑ chicken broth
- ❑ pickled jalapeño peppers
- ❑ pumpkin puree, unflavored
- ❑ tomato paste

Dairy Products
- ❑ bleu cheese, crumbled
- ❑ butter
- ❑ cheddar cheese
- ❑ cream cheese, low-fat
- ❑ Fontina cheese
- ❑ margarine, light
- ❑ milk, skim
- ❑ mozzarella cheese
- ❑ Parmigiano-Reggiano cheese
- ❑ Ricotta cheese, part-skim
- ❑ sour cream, reduced-fat
- ❑ yogurt, plain low-fat

Juice
- ❑ lime juice

Frozen Foods
- ❑ blueberries
- ❑ waffles, whole-grain

Meat and Poultry
- ❑ bacon
- ❑ chicken breast halves, skinless, bone-in
- ❑ chicken breast tenders
- ❑ eggs
- ❑ sea scallops
- ❑ steak strips, round tip
- ❑ turkey
- ❑ turkey bacon

Second Week Meals and Recipes

DAY 1

Breakfast

Waffles with Blueberry Maple Syrup

⅓ cup frozen blueberries   2 whole-grain waffles
2 tsp. maple syrup   1 tbsp. pecans

Microwave blueberries and syrup together for 2 to 3 minutes, until berries are thawed. Toast the waffles, top with warm blueberry syrup, and sprinkle with pecans. Serve with 1 cup skim milk. Serves 1.

Nutritional Information: 305 calories; 14g fat (42% calories from fat); 8g protein; 41g carbohydrate; 4g dietary fiber; 12mg cholesterol; 487mg sodium.

Lunch

Southwestern Cheese Panini

4 oz. shredded sharp cheddar cheese   1 tbsp. chopped pickled jalapeno
1 cup shredded zucchini   pepper (optional)
½ cup shredded carrot   8 slices whole-wheat bread
¼ cup finely chopped red onion   2 tsp. canola oil
¼ cup prepared salsa

Set aside four 15-ounce cans and a medium skillet (not nonstick) by the stove. Combine cheddar cheese, zucchini, carrots, onion, salsa and jalapenos (if using) in a medium bowl. Divide among 4 slices of bread and top with the remaining bread. Heat 1 teaspoon canola oil in a large nonstick skillet over medium heat and then place 2 of the panini in the pan. Place the medium skillet on top of the panini, and then weigh it down with the cans. Cook the panini until it is golden brown on one side (about 2 minutes). Reduce the heat to medium-low, flip the panini, replace the top skillet and cans, and then cook until the second side is also golden brown (about 1 to 3 minutes more). Repeat with another 1 teaspoon oil and the remaining panini. Serve with baby carrots with light Ranch dip. Serves 4.

Nutritional Information: 331 calories; 14g fat (38% calories from fat); 16g protein; 37g carbohydrate; 5g dietary fiber; 30mg cholesterol; 523mg sodium.

Dinner

Deviled Chicken

4 (8-oz.) skinless, bone-in chicken breast halves	2 tbsp. prepared mustard
½ tsp. freshly ground black pepper	½ tsp. ground red pepper
¼ tsp. salt	2 (1-oz.) slices French bread baguette
	nonstick cooking spray

Preheat oven to 475° F. Sprinkle chicken with black pepper and salt, and then lightly coat with the nonstick cooking spray. Place the chicken on the rack of a broiler or roasting pan coated with nonstick cooking spray. Bake at 475° F for 15 minutes, and then remove the pan from the oven. Combine mustard and red pepper in a small bowl and brush over the chicken. Place the bread in a food processor and pulse 10 times or until the crumbs measure 1 cup. Sprinkle breadcrumbs evenly over the mustard mixture on chicken, pressing lightly to adhere. Lightly coat breadcrumbs with nonstick cooking spray and return the pan to the oven. Bake at 475° F for 10 minutes or until breadcrumbs are browned and a thermometer inserted into the chicken registers 165° F. Serve with *Broccoli with Shallots* and *Herbed Rice*. Serves 4.

Nutritional Information: 214 calories; 4g fat (18% calories from fat); 34g protein; 9g carbohydrate; 0g dietary fiber; 90mg cholesterol; 408mg sodium.

Broccoli with Shallots

12 oz. fresh broccoli florets	2 tbsp. minced shallots
1 tsp. butter	¼ tsp. salt
1 tsp. olive oil	¼ tsp. black pepper

Cook the broccoli florets in boiling water for 2 minutes, and then drain. Heat the butter and olive oil in a skillet over medium-high heat. Add minced shallots and sauté for 2 minutes. Add broccoli, salt and black pepper and sauté for 2 minutes. Serves 4.

Nutritional Information: 38 calories; 2g fat (47% calories from fat); 2g protein; 4g carbohydrate; 2g dietary fiber; 3mg cholesterol; 25mg sodium.

Herbed Rice

1 cup basmati rice	½ tsp. cracked black pepper
1 tbsp. fresh thyme, chopped	⅜ tsp. salt
1 tsp. fresh oregano, chopped	

Cook basmati rice according to package directions. Stir in thyme, oregano, black pepper and salt. Serves 4.

Nutritional Information: 157 calories; 1g fat (6% calories from fat); 4g protein; 33g carbohydrate; trace dietary fiber; 0mg cholesterol; 31mg sodium.

DAY 2

....

Breakfast

Spinach and Bacon Omelet

1 egg plus 2 egg whites	1 slice whole-grain toast
2 slices turkey bacon, crumbled	1 tsp. butter
1 cup baby spinach	nonstick cooking spray

Whisk together eggs, bacon and spinach. Coat a skillet with nonstick cooking spray. Cook the egg mixture and serve with toast and butter.

Nutritional Information: 308 calories; 16g fat (46% calories from fat), 24g protein; 16g carbohydrate, 2g dietary fiber; 215mg cholesterol; 219mg sodium.

....

Lunch

Bleu Cheese and Beef Roll-ups

⅓ cup fat-free mayonnaise	⅛ tsp. salt
2 tbsp. crumbled bleu cheese	4 cups finely chopped romaine lettuce
½ tsp. prepared horseradish	1 cup halved grape tomatoes
¼ tsp. freshly ground black pepper, divided	¼ cup thinly sliced red onion
½ lb. round tip steak strips	4 (10-inch) reduced-fat flour tortillas
	nonstick cooking spray

Combine mayonnaise, bleu cheese, horseradish and ⅛ teaspoon black pepper in a small bowl, and then cover and refrigerate for 30 minutes. Heat a large nonstick skillet over medium-high heat. Coat a pan with nonstick cooking spray and sprinkle the steak with salt and the remaining ⅛ teaspoon pepper. Add the steak to the pan and sauté for 4 minutes or until desired degree of doneness. Let the steak stand for 5 minutes, and then cut into 1-inch pieces. Combine the lettuce, tomatoes and onion in a bowl. Spread about 2 tablespoons of the mayonnaise mixture evenly over each tortilla. Divide the steak and lettuce mixture evenly among tortillas and roll up. Serves 4.

Nutritional Information: 281 calories; 5g fat (16% calories from fat); 20g protein; 38g carbohydrate; 5g dietary fiber; 36mg cholesterol; 763mg sodium.

Dinner

Single serving egg-drop or wonton soup

Appetizer-size beef and broccoli or

chicken lettuce wraps (or split entrée version)

½ cup steamed or brown rice

Order the above items at a Chinese restaurant of your choice. Serves 1.

Nutritional Information: 494 calories; 10g fat (17.5% calories from fat); 18g protein; 83g carbohydrate; 6g dietary fiber; 25mg cholesterol; 517mg sodium.

DAY 3

Breakfast

Pumpkin and Granola Parfait

1 container (6-oz.) plain lowfat yogurt

2 tsp. honey

¼ tsp. pumpkin-pie spice

1 whole-grain crunchy granola bar, crumbled

½ cup canned pumpkin

Mix together yogurt, honey and pumpkin-pie spice. In a bowl, layer the yogurt mixture, granola-bar crumbs and pumpkin. Serves 1.

Nutritional Information: 304 calories; 5g fat (15% calories from fat); 8g protein; 55g carbohydrate; 5g dietary fiber; 0mg cholesterol; 203mg sodium.

Lunch

Seared Scallops with Pumpkin Soup

12 oz. fresh sea scallops

1 can (15-oz.) unflavored pumpkin puree

2 tbsp. roughly chopped hazelnuts

8 to 10 chives, chopped

1 cup chicken broth

1 tbsp. honey

1 tbsp. unsalted butter

½ tbsp. extra-virgin olive oil

Toast chopped hazelnuts in the oven (10 minutes at 400° F) or on the stove in a stainless steel saute pan (5 to 7 minutes over medium heat, shaking often so they don't burn). Set the hazelnuts aside. Combine pumpkin, honey, butter and broth in a medium saucepan and heat the mixture on low until it is warmed through. Season the mixture with salt and pepper to taste, and keep it warm. Next, preheat a cast-iron skillet or saute pan over medium-high heat. Pat scallops dry with a paper towel and season them with salt and pepper to taste. Add oil to the pan, and then add the scallops. Cook for 2 to 3 minutes on each side until they are firm, browned and caramelized. Pour the soup into wide-rimmed serving bowls. Add scallops and hazelnuts, and garnish with chopped chives. Serves 2.

Nutritional Information: 430 calories; 17g fat (36% calories from fat); 35g protein; 35g carbohydrate; 7g dietary fiber; 215mg cholesterol; 460mg sodium.

....

Dinner

Pan-Fried Chicken Fingers with Spicy Dipping Sauce

¼ cup canola mayonnaise	2 large eggs, lightly beaten
2 tsp. hot chili sauce	1 tbsp. water
1 tsp. fresh lime juice	3 cups whole-grain flake cereal
½ tsp. low-sodium soy sauce	1 lb. chicken breast tenders
¼ cup all-purpose flour	¼ tsp. salt
1½ tsp. freshly ground black pepper	1½ tbsp. canola oil
1½ tsp. paprika	

To prepare sauce, combine the mayonnaise, chili sauce, lime juice and soy sauce in a small bowl, stirring with a whisk. Cover and chill. To prepare the chicken, combine the flour, black pepper and paprika and place the mixture in a shallow dish. Combine eggs and 1 tablespoon water, and place in another shallow dish. Place the crushed cereal in another shallow dish. Sprinkle the chicken evenly with salt and then, working with 1 piece at a time, dredge the chicken in the flour mixture. Dip the chicken in the egg mixture, and then dredge in the cereal. Next, heat a large skillet over medium-high heat. Add oil to the pan, swirling to coat. Add chicken pieces to pan, and cook for 2 minutes on each side or until done. Serve immediately with sauce. Serves 4.

Nutritional Information: 414 calories; 14g fat (31% calories from fat); 34g protein; 38g carbohydrate; 4.5g dietary fiber; 156mg cholesterol; 495mg sodium.

DAY 4

....

Breakfast

Bagel with Cream Cheese and Tomato

1 small (3-oz.) whole-grain bagel
2 tbsp. lowfat cream cheese

2 large slices tomato
salt and pepper, to taste

Toast bagel halves and spread with cream cheese. Top each side with a slice of tomato and season with salt and pepper. Serve with 1 cup berries and 1 cup skim milk. Serves 1.

Nutritional Information: 302 calories; 7g fat (22% calories from fat); 13g protein; 52g carbohydrate; 8g dietary fiber; 0mg cholesterol; 7mg sodium.

....

Lunch

Black Bean Salad

2 cups chopped romaine lettuce
  hearts
1 avocado, chopped
1 medium tomato, chopped
½ cup canned black beans, rinsed
2 tbsp. diced green onion

1 tbsp. diced fresh cilantro
1 tbsp. olive oil
2 tsp. lime juice
¼ tsp. lime zest
¼ tsp. salt
½ tsp. ground black pepper

In a large bowl, toss together lettuce, avocado, tomato, beans, green onion and cilantro. In a small bowl, mix olive oil, lime juice, lime zest, salt and pepper. Pour dressing over the salad and toss well to coat. Serve with baked tortilla chips and fruit salad. Serves 2.

Nutritional Information: 247 calories; 17g fat (52% calories from fat); 6g protein; 20g carbohydrate; 9g dietary fiber; 0mg cholesterol; 311mg sodium.

....

Dinner

Eggplant Parmesan

2 large eggs, lightly beaten
1 tbsp. water
2 cups whole-wheat panko (Japanese
  breadcrumbs)
½ cup (2 oz.) grated fresh Parmigiano-
  Reggiano cheese, divided

2 (1-lb.) eggplants, peeled and cut
  crosswise into ½-inch thick slices
nonstick cooking spray
½ cup torn fresh basil
½ tsp. crushed red pepper
1½ tsp. minced garlic

⅜ tsp. salt
1 (16-oz.) container part-skim ricotta
cheese
1 large egg, lightly beaten
1 (24-oz.) jar premium pasta sauce

8 oz. thinly sliced mozzarella cheese
¾ cup (3 oz.) finely grated fontina
cheese

Preheat oven to 375° F. To make the eggplant, combine 2 eggs and 1 table-spoon water in a shallow dish. Combine panko and ¼ cup Parmigiano-Reggiano cheese in a second shallow dish. Dip the eggplant in the egg mixture and then dredge in the panko mixture, pressing gently to adhere and shaking off excess. Next, place the eggplants 1 inch apart on baking sheets coated with nonstick cooking spray. Bake at 375° F for 30 minutes or until golden, turning once and rotating the baking sheets after 15 minutes.

To make the filling, combine the basil, ¼ cup Parmigiano-Reggiano cheese, red pepper, minced garlic, ¼ teaspoon salt, ricotta cheese and egg. Spoon ½ cup of the pasta sauce into the bottom of a 13″ x 9″ glass baking dish coated with nonstick cooking spray. Layer half of eggplant slices over pasta sauce and sprinkle with ⅛ teaspoon salt. Top with about ¾ cup of the pasta sauce. Spread half of ricotta mixture over the sauce and top with a third of the mozzarella and ¼ cup fontina cheese. Repeat layers once, ending with about 1 cup of the pasta sauce.

Cover the eggplants tightly with aluminum foil coated with non-stick cooking spray. Bake at 375° F for 35 minutes. Remove the foil and top the eggplant with the remaining third of the mozzarella and ¼ cup fontina cheese. Bake at 375° F for 10 minutes or until the sauce is bub-bly and the cheese melts. Cool for 10 minutes. Serve with mixed green salad with light Ranch dressing and a breadstick. Serves 10.

Nutritional Information: 318 calories; 15g fat (48% calories from fat); 19g protein; 27g car-bohydrate; 5g dietary fiber; 99mg cholesterol; 65mg sodium.

DAY 5

Breakfast

Vanilla Spice French Toast with Apple

1 egg
2 egg whites

1 tsp. vanilla extract
dash of cinnamon

dash of nutmeg   ½ medium apple, sliced
2 pieces whole-grain bread

Whisk eggs, vanilla extract and cinnamon and nutmeg together. Dip the
bread into the egg mixture. Spray a skillet with nonstick cooking spray and
saute bread on each side until brown (about 3 minutes). Top with apple
slices. Serve with 1 cup skim milk. Serves 1.

Nutritional Information: 359 calories; 8g fat (20% calories from fat); 21g protein; 52g carbohydrate; 8g dietary fiber; 187mg cholesterol; 608mg sodium.

....

Lunch

Lo Mein Take Out

2 cups Chinese beef or chicken   ½ cup steamed vegetables
  lo mein   1 cup cubed pineapple

Nutritional Information: 401 calories; 14g fat (30% calories from fat); 26g protein; 45g carbohydrate; 3g dietary fiber; 25mg cholesterol; 1,280mg sodium.

....

Dinner

Glazed Scallops with Couscous

2½ tbsp. low-sodium soy sauce   1 cup fat-free, less-sodium chicken
1 tbsp. dark sesame oil   broth
2 tbsp. fresh lime juice   2 cups snow peas
2 tbsp. honey   1 cup packaged matchstick-cut carrots
¼ tsp. crushed red pepper   ¼ tsp. salt
16 large sea scallops (about 1½ lbs.) ¼ cup chopped fresh cilantro
½ cup uncooked couscous   (optional)

In a medium bowl, combine soy sauce, sesame oil, lime juice, honey and red
pepper. Rinse scallops under cold water and pat dry. Add scallops to marinade and toss well to coat. Let stand for 10 to 30 minutes, stirring once.
Next, bring the broth to a boil in a medium saucepan over high heat. Reduce
heat and stir in couscous, peas, carrots and salt. Cover and turn off heat,
and let stand 5 minutes. Meanwhile, prepare the grill and grill the scallops
over medium-hot coals for 3 minutes per side or until golden brown and
opaque in the center. Arrange the couscous mixture on 4 plates and then
arrange 4 scallops over the couscous. Bring the marinade to a boil, stir and

cook for 3 minutes or until thickened. Drizzle the mixture over the scallops and couscous and top with cilantro, if desired. Serve with 1 whole-grain dinner roll. Serves 4.

Nutritional Information: 335 calories; 5g fat (22% calories from fat); 34g protein; 37g carbohydrate; 3g dietary fiber; 56mg cholesterol; 740mg sodium.

DAY 6

....

Breakfast

Honey and Pear Oatmeal with Almonds

· 1 medium pear, diced
2 tsp. honey

1 packet instant plain oatmeal
1 tbsp. almonds, chopped

Microwave the pear and honey until warm (about 3 minutes). Prepare the oatmeal with hot water and top with pear and honey. Sprinkle with almonds. Serves 1.

Nutritional Information: 492 calories; 10g fat (18% calories from fat); 15g protein; 90g carbohydrate; 14g dietary fiber; 0mg cholesterol; 820mg sodium.

....

Lunch

Fresh Tomato Soup

2 cups fat-free, less-sodium chicken broth
1 cup chopped onion
¾ cup chopped celery
1 tbsp. thinly sliced fresh basil
1 tbsp. tomato paste

2 lbs. plum tomatoes, cut into wedges
½ tsp. salt
¼ tsp. freshly ground black pepper
6 tbsp. plain lowfat yogurt
3 tbsp. thinly sliced fresh basil

Combine chicken broth, onion, celery, basil, tomato paste and tomatoes in a large saucepan and bring to a boil. Reduce heat and simmer 30 minutes. Place half of the tomato mixture in a blender. Remove the center piece of the blender lid (to allow steam to escape) and secure the blender lid on the blender. Place a clean towel over the opening in the blender lid (to avoid splatters) and blend until smooth. Pour the mixture into a large bowl and repeat the procedure with the remaining tomato mixture. Stir in salt and pepper. Ladle ¾ cup soup into each of 6 bowls and top each serving with 1 tablespoon yogurt and 1½ teaspoons basil. Serve with ½ turkey sandwich on whole-grain bread with light mayo or Dijon mustard, lettuce and tomato. Serves 6.

Nutritional Information: 58 calories; 1g fat (12% calories from fat); 3g protein; 11g carbohydrate; 3g dietary fiber; 1mg cholesterol; 382mg sodium.

....

Dinner

Taco Bell Fresco Style Crunchy   1 serving Mexican Rice
  Taco®

Nutritional Information: 511 calories; 18g fat (32% calories from fat); 16g protein; 68g carbohydrate; 11g dietary fiber; 40mg cholesterol; 1,110mg sodium.

DAY 7

....

Breakfast

Takeout from Jamba Juice®   16-oz. Protein Berry Workout®

Nutritional Information: 280 calories; 0g fat (0% calories from fat); 17g protein; 52g carbohydrate; 3g dietary fiber; 5mg cholesterol; 115mg sodium.

....

Lunch

Salad BLTs

¼ cup fat-free mayonnaise
3 tbsp. thinly sliced green onions
3 tbsp. reduced-fat sour cream
2 tsp. whole-grain Dijon mustard
½ tsp. freshly ground black pepper
¼ tsp. grated lemon rind
8 hard-cooked large eggs

8 (1½-oz.) slices peasant bread or
  firm sandwich bread, toasted
4 center-cut bacon slices, cooked and
  cut in half crosswise
8 (¼-inch-thick) slices tomato
4 large Boston lettuce leaves

Combine mayonnaise, onions, sour cream, Dijon mustard, pepper and lemon rind in a medium bowl, stirring well. Cut 2 eggs in half lengthwise, and reserve the yolks for another use. Coarsely chop the remaining egg whites and whole eggs. Add eggs to the mayonnaise mixture and stir gently to combine. Next, arrange 4 bread slices on a cutting board or work surface. Top each bread slice with ½ cup of the egg mixture, 2 bacon pieces, 2 tomato slices, 1 lettuce leaf and 1 bread slice. Serve with baked chips and an orange. Serves 4.

Nutritional Information: 371 calories; 12g fat (29% calories from fat); 22g protein; 44g carbohydrate; 2g dietary fiber; 329mg cholesterol; 892mg sodium.

....

Dinner

Easy Shrimp Fettucini Alfredo

1 package reduced-fat cream cheese
¼ cup Parmesan cheese
½ cup skim milk

2 tbsp. light margarine
salt and pepper, to taste

Combine all ingredients in a small saucepan. Heat over low heat, stirring frequently until cheese has melted. Pour over hot noodles. Serve with mixed green salad with light dressing and a whole-grain dinner roll. Serves 2.

Nutritional Information: 362 calories; 14g fat (34% calories from fat); 15g protein; 44g carbohydrate; 2g dietary fiber; 70mg cholesterol; 447mg sodium.

HEALTHY SNACK OPTIONS

(**Note:** You will need to add the ingredients for each of these items to the grocery lists. All are less than 100 calories!)

- ½ cup of sugar-free gelatin, any flavor, and two tablespoons of low-fat Cool Whip®
- 2 teaspoons of Hershey's chocolate syrup in a cup of coffee (makes a great café mocha!)
- ¼ cup fat-free Ranch dressing and 1 cup of mixed fresh veggies, such as jicama, red bell pepper, celery, carrot sticks or cherry tomatoes
- 6 saltine crackers and 2 teaspoons of peanut butter
- marshmallow on top of a graham cracker, microwaved until gooey, with a teaspoon of Hershey's chocolate syrup drizzled over the top
- ½ an apple with 2 teaspoons of peanut butter
- ½ cup of frozen orange juice (nice little sorbet!)
- 2 graham cracker squares, spread with 1 teaspoon of peanut butter
- A cup of coffee and a small biscotti

ADDITIONAL RECIPES

Luscious Parfait

½ cup low-fat pudding   Cool Whip®
vanilla wafers, crumbled

Layer the pudding into a parfait glass, alternating with two crumbled vanilla wafers and a dollop of Cool Whip gracing the top. Serves 1.

Nutritional Information: 145 calories; 3.5g fat (22% calories from fat); 1g protein; 24g carbohydrate; 0g dietary fiber; 0mg cholesterol; 160mg sodium.

Salsa Potato

baked potato, small   2 tbsp. nonfat sour cream
½ cup salsa

Spoon the salsa and sour cream over the baked potato. Serves 1.

Nutritional Information: 95 calories; 0g fat (0% calories from fat); 3.1g protein; 16g carbohydrate; 0g dietary fiber; 9mg cholesterol; 141mg sodium.

Kettle Corn

½ tsp. paprika   ⅛ tsp. cayenne pepper
½ tsp. salt   5 tbsp. sugar
¼ tsp. ground coriander   1 tbsp. butter
¼ tsp. white pepper

Mix paprika, salt, ground coriander, white pepper and cayenne pepper in a bowl. Make a bag of low-fat microwave popcorn. While it pops, cook the sugar in a saucepan over medium heat until it melts and turns light brown. Remove the mixture from the heat and stir in the butter. Pour the caramel over the popcorn in a bowl, sprinkle with the spice mix and toss. Spread out on a baking sheet to cool. Serves 2 (1-cup servings).

Nutritional Information: 225 calories; 7g fat (27% calories from fat); 3.5g protein; 50g carbohydrate; 4g dietary fiber; 15mg cholesterol; 700mg sodium.

Member Survey

Please answer the following questions to help your leader plan your First Place 4 Health meetings so that your needs might be met in this session. Give this form to your leader at the first group meeting.

Name _____ Birth date _____

Please list those who live in your household.

Name	Relationship	Age

What church do you attend? _____

Are you interested in receiving more information about our church?

      Yes   No

Occupation _____

What talent or area of expertise would you be willing to share with our class?

_____

Why did you join First Place 4 Health?

_____

With notice, would you be willing to lead a Bible study discussion one week?

      Yes   No

Are you comfortable praying out loud? _____

If the assistant leader were absent, would you be willing to assist in weighing in members and possibly evaluating the Live It Trackers?

      Yes   No

Any other comments:

_____

_____

Personal Weight and Measurement Record

Week	Weight	+ or -	Goal this Session	Pounds to goal
1				
2				
3				
4				
5				
6				
7				
8				
9				
10				
11				
12				

Beginning Measurements

Waist _____ Hips _____ Thighs _____ Chest _____

Ending Measurements

Waist _____ Hips _____ Thighs _____ Chest _____

First Place 4 Health
Prayer Partner

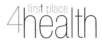

A NEW
BEGINNING
Week
1

Scripture Verse to Memorize for Week Two:

*Therefore, if anyone is in Christ, he is a new creation;
the old has gone, the new has come!*

2 Corinthians 5:17

Date: _____

Name: _____

Home Phone: (_____) _____

Work Phone: (_____) _____

Email: _____

Personal Prayer Concerns:

_____

_____

_____

_____

_____

_____

_____

This form is for prayer requests that are personal to you and your journey in First Place 4 Health. Please complete this form and have it ready to turn in when you arrive at your group meeting.

First Place 4 Health
Prayer Partner

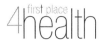

SCRIPTURE VERSE TO MEMORIZE FOR WEEK THREE:

*And we know that in all things God works for the good of those who love him,
who have been called according to his purpose.*

ROMANS 8:28

Date: _____

Name: _____

Home Phone: (_____) _____

Work Phone: (_____) _____

Email: _____

Personal Prayer Concerns:

_____

_____

_____

_____

_____

_____

_____

This form is for prayer requests that are personal to you and your journey in First Place 4 Health. Please complete this form and have it ready to turn in when you arrive at your group meeting.

First Place 4 Health
Prayer Partner

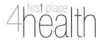

A NEW
BEGINNING
Week
3

SCRIPTURE VERSE TO MEMORIZE FOR WEEK FOUR:

He has showed you, O man, what is good. And what does the LORD require of you?
To act justly and to love mercy and to walk humbly with your God.

MICAH 6:8

Date: _____

Name: _____

Home Phone: (_____) _____

Work Phone: (_____) _____

Email: _____

Personal Prayer Concerns:

_____

_____

_____

_____

_____

_____

_____

This form is for prayer requests that are personal to you and your journey in First Place 4 Health. Please complete this form and have it ready to turn in when you arrive at your group meeting.

First Place 4 Health
Prayer Partner

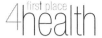

SCRIPTURE VERSE TO MEMORIZE FOR WEEK FIVE:

*But he said to me, "My grace is sufficient for you, for my power is
made perfect in weakness." Therefore I will boast all the more gladly about
my weaknesses, so that Christ's power may rest on me.*

2 CORINTHIANS 12:9

Date: _____

Name: _____

Home Phone: (_____) _____

Work Phone: (_____) _____

Email: _____

Personal Prayer Concerns:

_____

_____

_____

_____

_____

_____

_____

This form is for prayer requests that are personal to you and your journey in First Place 4 Health. Please complete this
form and have it ready to turn in when you arrive at your group meeting.

First Place 4 Health
Prayer Partner

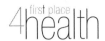

SCRIPTURE VERSE TO MEMORIZE FOR WEEK SIX:

Being confident of this, that he who began a good work in you will carry it on to completion until the day of Christ Jesus.

PHILIPPIANS 1:6

Date: _____

Name: _____

Home Phone: (_____) _____

Work Phone: (_____) _____

Email: _____

Personal Prayer Concerns:

_____

_____

_____

_____

_____

_____

_____

This form is for prayer requests that are personal to you and your journey in First Place 4 Health. Please complete this form and have it ready to turn in when you arrive at your group meeting.

First Place 4 Health
Prayer Partner

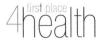

A NEW
BEGINNING
Week
6

SCRIPTURE VERSE TO MEMORIZE FOR WEEK SEVEN:

Whatever you do, work at it with all your heart, as working for the Lord, not for men.

COLOSSIANS 3:23

Date: _____

Name: _____

Home Phone: (_____) _____

Work Phone: (_____) _____

Email: _____

Personal Prayer Concerns:

_____

_____

_____

_____

_____

_____

_____

This form is for prayer requests that are personal to you and your journey in First Place 4 Health. Please complete this form and have it ready to turn in when you arrive at your group meeting.

First Place 4 Health
Prayer Partner

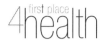

SCRIPTURE VERSE TO MEMORIZE FOR WEEK EIGHT:

From the fullness of his grace we have all received one blessing after another.

JOHN 1:16

Date: _____

Name: _____

Home Phone: (_____)_____

Work Phone: (_____)_____

Email: _____

Personal Prayer Concerns:

_____

_____

_____

_____

_____

_____

_____

This form is for prayer requests that are personal to you and your journey in First Place 4 Health. Please complete this form and have it ready to turn in when you arrive at your group meeting.

First Place 4 Health
Prayer Partner

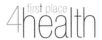

SCRIPTURE VERSE TO MEMORIZE FOR WEEK NINE:

That at the name of Jesus every knee should bow, in heaven and on earth and under the earth, and every tongue confess that Jesus Christ is Lord, to the glory of God the Father.

PHILIPPIANS 2:10-11

Date: _____

Name: _____

Home Phone: (_____) _____

Work Phone: (_____) _____

Email: _____

Personal Prayer Concerns:

_____

_____

_____

_____

_____

_____

_____

This form is for prayer requests that are personal to you and your journey in First Place 4 Health. Please complete this form and have it ready to turn in when you arrive at your group meeting.

First Place 4 Health
Prayer Partner

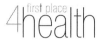

A NEW
BEGINNING
Week
9

SCRIPTURE VERSE TO MEMORIZE FOR WEEK TEN:

No one will be able to stand up against you all the days of your life. As I was with Moses, so I will be with you; I will never leave you nor forsake you.

JOSHUA 1:5

Date: _____

Name: _____

Home Phone: (_____)_____

Work Phone: (_____)_____

Email: _____

Personal Prayer Concerns:

_____

_____

_____

_____

_____

_____

_____

This form is for prayer requests that are personal to you and your journey in First Place 4 Health. Please complete this form and have it ready to turn in when you arrive at your group meeting.

First Place 4 Health
Prayer Partner

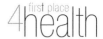

A NEW
BEGINNING
Week
10

Date: _____

Name: _____

Home Phone: (_____)_____

Work Phone: (_____)_____

Email: _____

Personal Prayer Concerns:

_____

_____

_____

_____

_____

_____

_____

This form is for prayer requests that are personal to you and your journey in First Place 4 Health. Please complete this form and have it ready to turn in when you arrive at your group meeting.

First Place 4 Health
Prayer Partner

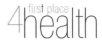

A NEW
BEGINNING
Week
11

Date: _____

Name: _____

Home Phone: (____) _____

Work Phone: (____) _____

Email: _____

Personal Prayer Concerns:

_____

_____

_____

_____

_____

_____

_____

This form is for prayer requests that are personal to you and your journey in First Place 4 Health. Please complete this form and have it ready to turn in when you arrive at your group meeting.

Live It Tracker

Name: _____ Loss/gain: _____ lbs.

Date: _____ Week #: _____ Calorie Range: _____ My food goal for next week: _____

Activity Level: None, < 30 min/day, 30-60 min/day, 60+ min/day My activity goal for next week: _____

Group	Daily Calories							
	1300-1400	1500-1600	1700-1800	1900-2000	2100-2200	2300-2400	2500-2600	2700-2800
Fruits	1.5-2 c.	1.5-2 c.	1.5-2 c.	2-2.5 c.	2-2.5 c.	2.5-3.5 c.	3.5-4.5 c.	3.5-4.5 c.
Vegetables	1.5-2 c.	2-2.5 c.	2.5-3 c.	2.5-3 c.	3-3.5 c.	3.5-4.5 c.	4.5-5 c.	4.5-5 c.
Grains	5 oz-eq.	5-6 oz-eq.	6-7 oz-eq.	6-7 oz-eq.	7-8 oz-eq.	8-9 oz-eq.	9-10 oz-eq.	10-11 oz-eq.
Meat & Beans	4 oz-eq.	5 oz-eq.	5-5.5 oz-eq.	5.5-6.5 oz-eq.	6.5-7 oz-eq.	7-7.5 oz-eq.	7-7.5 oz-eq.	7.5-8 oz-eq.
Milk	2-3 c.	3 c.	3 c.	3 c.	3 c.	3 c.	3 c.	3 c.
Healthy Oils	4 tsp.	5 tsp.	5 tsp.	6 tsp.	6 tsp.	7 tsp.	8 tsp.	8 tsp.

Day/Date:

Breakfast: _____ Lunch: _____

Dinner: _____ Snack: _____

Group	Fruits	Vegetables	Grains	Meat & Beans	Milk	Oils
Goal Amount						
Estimate Your Total						
Increase ⇧ or Decrease? ⇩						

Physical Activity: _____ Spiritual Activity: _____

Steps/Miles/Minutes: _____ _____

Day/Date:

Breakfast: _____ Lunch: _____

Dinner: _____ Snack: _____

Group	Fruits	Vegetables	Grains	Meat & Beans	Milk	Oils
Goal Amount						
Estimate Your Total						
Increase ⇧ or Decrease? ⇩						

Physical Activity: _____ Spiritual Activity: _____

Steps/Miles/Minutes: _____ _____

Day/Date:

Breakfast: _____ Lunch: _____

Dinner: _____ Snack: _____

Group	Fruits	Vegetables	Grains	Meat & Beans	Milk	Oils
Goal Amount						
Estimate Your Total						
Increase ⇧ or Decrease? ⇩						

Physical Activity: _____ Spiritual Activity: _____

Steps/Miles/Minutes: _____ _____

Day/Date:

Breakfast: _____ Lunch: _____

Dinner: _____ Snack: _____

Group	Fruits	Vegetables	Grains	Meat & Beans	Milk	Oils
Goal Amount						
Estimate Your Total						
Increase ⇧ or Decrease? ⇩						

Physical Activity: _____ Spiritual Activity: _____

Steps/Miles/Minutes: _____ _____

Day/Date:

Breakfast: _____ Lunch: _____

Dinner: _____ Snack: _____

Group	Fruits	Vegetables	Grains	Meat & Beans	Milk	Oils
Goal Amount						
Estimate Your Total						
Increase ⇧ or Decrease? ⇩						

Physical Activity: _____ Spiritual Activity: _____

Steps/Miles/Minutes: _____ _____

Day/Date:

Breakfast: _____ Lunch: _____

Dinner: _____ Snack: _____

Group	Fruits	Vegetables	Grains	Meat & Beans	Milk	Oils
Goal Amount						
Estimate Your Total						
Increase ⇧ or Decrease? ⇩						

Physical Activity: _____ Spiritual Activity: _____

Steps/Miles/Minutes: _____ _____

Day/Date:

Breakfast: _____ Lunch: _____

Dinner: _____ Snack: _____

Group	Fruits	Vegetables	Grains	Meat & Beans	Milk	Oils
Goal Amount						
Estimate Your Total						
Increase ⇧ or Decrease? ⇩						

Physical Activity: _____ Spiritual Activity: _____

Steps/Miles/Minutes: _____ _____

Live It Tracker

Name: _____ Loss/gain: _____ lbs.

Date: _____ Week #: _____ Calorie Range: _____ My food goal for next week: _____

Activity Level: None, < 30 min/day, 30-60 min/day, 60+ min/day My activity goal for next week: _____

Group	Daily Calories							
	1300-1400	1500-1600	1700-1800	1900-2000	2100-2200	2300-2400	2500-2600	2700-2800
Fruits	1.5-2 c.	1.5-2 c.	1.5-2 c.	2-2.5 c.	2-2.5 c.	2.5-3.5 c.	3.5-4.5 c.	3.5-4.5 c.
Vegetables	1.5-2 c.	2-2.5 c.	2.5-3 c.	2.5-3 c.	3-3.5 c.	3.5-4.5 c.	4.5-5 c.	4.5-5 c.
Grains	5 oz-eq.	5-6 oz-eq.	6-7 oz-eq.	6-7 oz-eq.	7-8 oz-eq.	8-9 oz-eq.	9-10 oz-eq.	10-11 oz-eq.
Meat & Beans	4 oz-eq.	5 oz-eq.	5-5.5 oz-eq.	5.5-6.5 oz-eq.	6.5-7 oz-eq.	7-7.5 oz-eq.	7-7.5 oz-eq.	7.5-8 oz-eq.
Milk	2-3 c.	3 c.	3 c.	3 c.	3 c.	3 c.	3 c.	3 c.
Healthy Oils	4 tsp.	5 tsp.	5 tsp.	6 tsp.	6 tsp.	7 tsp.	8 tsp.	8 tsp.

Day/Date: _____

Breakfast: _____ Lunch: _____

Dinner: _____ Snack: _____

Group	Fruits	Vegetables	Grains	Meat & Beans	Milk	Oils
Goal Amount						
Estimate Your Total						
Increase ⇧ or Decrease? ⇩						

Physical Activity: _____ Spiritual Activity: _____

Steps/Miles/Minutes: _____

Day/Date: _____

Breakfast: _____ Lunch: _____

Dinner: _____ Snack: _____

Group	Fruits	Vegetables	Grains	Meat & Beans	Milk	Oils
Goal Amount						
Estimate Your Total						
Increase ⇧ or Decrease? ⇩						

Physical Activity: _____ Spiritual Activity: _____

Steps/Miles/Minutes: _____

Day/Date: _____

Breakfast: _____ Lunch: _____

Dinner: _____ Snack: _____

Group	Fruits	Vegetables	Grains	Meat & Beans	Milk	Oils
Goal Amount						
Estimate Your Total						
Increase ⇧ or Decrease? ⇩						

Physical Activity: _____ Spiritual Activity: _____

Steps/Miles/Minutes: _____

Day/Date:

Breakfast: _____   Lunch: _____

Dinner: _____   Snack: _____

Group	Fruits	Vegetables	Grains	Meat & Beans	Milk	Oils
Goal Amount						
Estimate Your Total						
Increase ⇧ or Decrease? ⇩						

Physical Activity: _____   Spiritual Activity: _____

Steps/Miles/Minutes: _____   _____

Day/Date:

Breakfast: _____   Lunch: _____

Dinner: _____   Snack: _____

Group	Fruits	Vegetables	Grains	Meat & Beans	Milk	Oils
Goal Amount						
Estimate Your Total						
Increase ⇧ or Decrease? ⇩						

Physical Activity: _____   Spiritual Activity: _____

Steps/Miles/Minutes: _____   _____

Day/Date:

Breakfast: _____   Lunch: _____

Dinner: _____   Snack: _____

Group	Fruits	Vegetables	Grains	Meat & Beans	Milk	Oils
Goal Amount						
Estimate Your Total						
Increase ⇧ or Decrease? ⇩						

Physical Activity: _____   Spiritual Activity: _____

Steps/Miles/Minutes: _____   _____

Day/Date:

Breakfast: _____   Lunch: _____

Dinner: _____   Snack: _____

Group	Fruits	Vegetables	Grains	Meat & Beans	Milk	Oils
Goal Amount						
Estimate Your Total						
Increase ⇧ or Decrease? ⇩						

Physical Activity: _____   Spiritual Activity: _____

Steps/Miles/Minutes: _____   _____

Live It Tracker

Name: _____ Loss/gain: _____ lbs.

Date: _____ Week #: ____ Calorie Range: _____ My food goal for next week: _____

Activity Level: None, < 30 min/day, 30-60 min/day, 60+ min/day My activity goal for next week: _____

Group	Daily Calories							
	1300-1400	1500-1600	1700-1800	1900-2000	2100-2200	2300-2400	2500-2600	2700-2800
Fruits	1.5-2 c.	1.5-2 c.	1.5-2 c.	2-2.5 c.	2-2.5 c.	2.5-3.5 c.	3.5-4.5 c.	3.5-4.5 c.
Vegetables	1.5-2 c.	2-2.5 c.	2.5-3 c.	2.5-3 c.	3-3.5 c.	3.5-4.5 c.	4.5-5 c.	4.5-5 c.
Grains	5 oz-eq.	5-6 oz-eq.	6-7 oz-eq.	6-7 oz-eq.	7-8 oz-eq.	8-9 oz-eq.	9-10 oz-eq.	10-11 oz-eq.
Meat & Beans	4 oz-eq.	5 oz-eq.	5-5.5 oz-eq.	5.5-6.5 oz-eq.	6.5-7 oz-eq.	7-7.5 oz-eq.	7-7.5 oz-eq.	7.5-8 oz-eq.
Milk	2-3 c.	3 c.	3 c.	3 c.	3 c.	3 c.	3 c.	3 c.
Healthy Oils	4 tsp.	5 tsp.	5 tsp.	6 tsp.	6 tsp.	7 tsp.	8 tsp.	8 tsp.

Day/Date: ____

Breakfast: _____ Lunch: _____

Dinner: _____ Snack: _____

Group	Fruits	Vegetables	Grains	Meat & Beans	Milk	Oils
Goal Amount						
Estimate Your Total						
Increase ⇧ or Decrease? ⇩						

Physical Activity: _____ Spiritual Activity: _____

Steps/Miles/Minutes: _____

Day/Date: ____

Breakfast: _____ Lunch: _____

Dinner: _____ Snack: _____

Group	Fruits	Vegetables	Grains	Meat & Beans	Milk	Oils
Goal Amount						
Estimate Your Total						
Increase ⇧ or Decrease? ⇩						

Physical Activity: _____ Spiritual Activity: _____

Steps/Miles/Minutes: _____

Day/Date: ____

Breakfast: _____ Lunch: _____

Dinner: _____ Snack: _____

Group	Fruits	Vegetables	Grains	Meat & Beans	Milk	Oils
Goal Amount						
Estimate Your Total						
Increase ⇧ or Decrease? ⇩						

Physical Activity: _____ Spiritual Activity: _____

Steps/Miles/Minutes: _____

Day/Date:

Breakfast: _____ Lunch: _____

Dinner: _____ Snack: _____

Group	Fruits	Vegetables	Grains	Meat & Beans	Milk	Oils
Goal Amount						
Estimate Your Total						
Increase ⇧ or Decrease? ⇩						

Physical Activity: _____ Spiritual Activity: _____

Steps/Miles/Minutes: _____ _____

Day/Date:

Breakfast: _____ Lunch: _____

Dinner: _____ Snack: _____

Group	Fruits	Vegetables	Grains	Meat & Beans	Milk	Oils
Goal Amount						
Estimate Your Total						
Increase ⇧ or Decrease? ⇩						

Physical Activity: _____ Spiritual Activity: _____

Steps/Miles/Minutes: _____ _____

Day/Date:

Breakfast: _____ Lunch: _____

Dinner: _____ Snack: _____

Group	Fruits	Vegetables	Grains	Meat & Beans	Milk	Oils
Goal Amount						
Estimate Your Total						
Increase ⇧ or Decrease? ⇩						

Physical Activity: _____ Spiritual Activity: _____

Steps/Miles/Minutes: _____ _____

Day/Date:

Breakfast: _____ Lunch: _____

Dinner: _____ Snack: _____

Group	Fruits	Vegetables	Grains	Meat & Beans	Milk	Oils
Goal Amount						
Estimate Your Total						
Increase ⇧ or Decrease? ⇩						

Physical Activity: _____ Spiritual Activity: _____

Steps/Miles/Minutes: _____ _____

Live It Tracker

Name: _____ Loss/gain: _____ lbs.

Date: _____ Week #: ____ Calorie Range: _____ My food goal for next week: _____

Activity Level: None, < 30 min/day, 30-60 min/day, 60+ min/day My activity goal for next week: _____

Group	Daily Calories							
	1300-1400	1500-1600	1700-1800	1900-2000	2100-2200	2300-2400	2500-2600	2700-2800
Fruits	1.5-2 c.	1.5-2 c.	1.5-2 c.	2-2.5 c.	2-2.5 c.	2.5-3.5 c.	3.5-4.5 c.	3.5-4.5 c.
Vegetables	1.5-2 c.	2-2.5 c.	2.5-3 c.	2.5-3 c.	3-3.5 c.	3.5-4.5 c.	4.5-5 c.	4.5-5 c.
Grains	5 oz-eq.	5-6 oz-eq.	6-7 oz-eq.	6-7 oz-eq.	7-8 oz-eq.	8-9 oz-eq.	9-10 oz-eq.	10-11 oz-eq.
Meat & Beans	4 oz-eq.	5 oz-eq.	5-5.5 oz-eq.	5.5-6.5 oz-eq.	6.5-7 oz-eq.	7-7.5 oz-eq.	7-7.5 oz-eq.	7.5-8 oz-eq.
Milk	2-3 c.	3 c.	3 c.	3 c.	3 c.	3 c.	3 c.	3 c.
Healthy Oils	4 tsp.	5 tsp.	5 tsp.	6 tsp.	6 tsp.	7 tsp.	8 tsp.	8 tsp.

Day/Date:

Breakfast: _____ Lunch: _____

Dinner: _____ Snack: _____

Group	Fruits	Vegetables	Grains	Meat & Beans	Milk	Oils
Goal Amount						
Estimate Your Total						
Increase ⇧ or Decrease? ⇩						

Physical Activity: _____ Spiritual Activity: _____

Steps/Miles/Minutes: _____ _____

Day/Date:

Breakfast: _____ Lunch: _____

Dinner: _____ Snack: _____

Group	Fruits	Vegetables	Grains	Meat & Beans	Milk	Oils
Goal Amount						
Estimate Your Total						
Increase ⇧ or Decrease? ⇩						

Physical Activity: _____ Spiritual Activity: _____

Steps/Miles/Minutes: _____ _____

Day/Date:

Breakfast: _____ Lunch: _____

Dinner: _____ Snack: _____

Group	Fruits	Vegetables	Grains	Meat & Beans	Milk	Oils
Goal Amount						
Estimate Your Total						
Increase ⇧ or Decrease? ⇩						

Physical Activity: _____ Spiritual Activity: _____

Steps/Miles/Minutes: _____ _____

Breakfast: _____ Lunch: _____

Dinner: _____ Snack: _____

Group	Fruits	Vegetables	Grains	Meat & Beans	Milk	Oils
Goal Amount						
Estimate Your Total						
Increase ⇧ or Decrease? ⇩						

Physical Activity: _____ Spiritual Activity: _____

Steps/Miles/Minutes: _____ _____

Day/Date: ___

Breakfast: _____ Lunch: _____

Dinner: _____ Snack: _____

Group	Fruits	Vegetables	Grains	Meat & Beans	Milk	Oils
Goal Amount						
Estimate Your Total						
Increase ⇧ or Decrease? ⇩						

Physical Activity: _____ Spiritual Activity: _____

Steps/Miles/Minutes: _____ _____

Day/Date: ___

Breakfast: _____ Lunch: _____

Dinner: _____ Snack: _____

Group	Fruits	Vegetables	Grains	Meat & Beans	Milk	Oils
Goal Amount						
Estimate Your Total						
Increase ⇧ or Decrease? ⇩						

Physical Activity: _____ Spiritual Activity: _____

Steps/Miles/Minutes: _____ _____

Day/Date: ___

Breakfast: _____ Lunch: _____

Dinner: _____ Snack: _____

Group	Fruits	Vegetables	Grains	Meat & Beans	Milk	Oils
Goal Amount						
Estimate Your Total						
Increase ⇧ or Decrease? ⇩						

Physical Activity: _____ Spiritual Activity: _____

Steps/Miles/Minutes: _____ _____

Day/Date: ___

Live It Tracker

Name: _____ Loss/gain: _____ lbs.

Date: _____ Week #: _____ Calorie Range: _____ My food goal for next week: _____

Activity Level: None, < 30 min/day, 30-60 min/day, 60+ min/day My activity goal for next week: _____

Group	Daily Calories							
	1300-1400	1500-1600	1700-1800	1900-2000	2100-2200	2300-2400	2500-2600	2700-2800
Fruits	1.5-2 c.	1.5-2 c.	1.5-2 c.	2-2.5 c.	2-2.5 c.	2.5-3.5 c.	3.5-4.5 c.	3.5-4.5 c.
Vegetables	1.5-2 c.	2-2.5 c.	2.5-3 c.	2.5-3 c.	3-3.5 c.	3.5-4.5 c.	4.5-5 c.	4.5-5 c.
Grains	5 oz-eq.	5-6 oz-eq.	6-7 oz-eq.	6-7 oz-eq.	7-8 oz-eq.	8-9 oz-eq.	9-10 oz-eq.	10-11 oz-eq.
Meat & Beans	4 oz-eq.	5 oz-eq.	5-5.5 oz-eq.	5.5-6.5 oz-eq.	6.5-7 oz-eq.	7-7.5 oz-eq.	7-7.5 oz-eq.	7.5-8 oz-eq.
Milk	2-3 c.	3 c.	3 c.	3 c.	3 c.	3 c.	3 c.	3 c.
Healthy Oils	4 tsp.	5 tsp.	5 tsp.	6 tsp.	6 tsp.	7 tsp.	8 tsp.	8 tsp.

Day/Date:

Breakfast: _____ Lunch: _____

Dinner: _____ Snack: _____

Group	Fruits	Vegetables	Grains	Meat & Beans	Milk	Oils
Goal Amount						
Estimate Your Total						
Increase ⇧ or Decrease? ⇩						

Physical Activity: _____ Spiritual Activity: _____

Steps/Miles/Minutes: _____

Day/Date:

Breakfast: _____ Lunch: _____

Dinner: _____ Snack: _____

Group	Fruits	Vegetables	Grains	Meat & Beans	Milk	Oils
Goal Amount						
Estimate Your Total						
Increase ⇧ or Decrease? ⇩						

Physical Activity: _____ Spiritual Activity: _____

Steps/Miles/Minutes: _____

Day/Date:

Breakfast: _____ Lunch: _____

Dinner: _____ Snack: _____

Group	Fruits	Vegetables	Grains	Meat & Beans	Milk	Oils
Goal Amount						
Estimate Your Total						
Increase ⇧ or Decrease? ⇩						

Physical Activity: _____ Spiritual Activity: _____

Steps/Miles/Minutes: _____

Day/Date: _____

Breakfast: _____ Lunch: _____

Dinner: _____ Snack: _____

Group	Fruits	Vegetables	Grains	Meat & Beans	Milk	Oils
Goal Amount						
Estimate Your Total						
Increase ⇧ or Decrease? ⇩						

Physical Activity: _____ Spiritual Activity: _____

Steps/Miles/Minutes: _____

Day/Date: _____

Breakfast: _____ Lunch: _____

Dinner: _____ Snack: _____

Group	Fruits	Vegetables	Grains	Meat & Beans	Milk	Oils
Goal Amount						
Estimate Your Total						
Increase ⇧ or Decrease? ⇩						

Physical Activity: _____ Spiritual Activity: _____

Steps/Miles/Minutes: _____

Day/Date: _____

Breakfast: _____ Lunch: _____

Dinner: _____ Snack: _____

Group	Fruits	Vegetables	Grains	Meat & Beans	Milk	Oils
Goal Amount						
Estimate Your Total						
Increase ⇧ or Decrease? ⇩						

Physical Activity: _____ Spiritual Activity: _____

Steps/Miles/Minutes: _____

Day/Date: _____

Breakfast: _____ Lunch: _____

Dinner: _____ Snack: _____

Group	Fruits	Vegetables	Grains	Meat & Beans	Milk	Oils
Goal Amount						
Estimate Your Total						
Increase ⇧ or Decrease? ⇩						

Physical Activity: _____ Spiritual Activity: _____

Steps/Miles/Minutes: _____

Live It Tracker

Name: _____ Loss/gain: _____ lbs.

Date: _____ Week #: _____ Calorie Range: _____ My food goal for next week: _____

Activity Level: None, < 30 min/day, 30-60 min/day, 60+ min/day My activity goal for next week: _____

Group	Daily Calories							
	1300-1400	1500-1600	1700-1800	1900-2000	2100-2200	2300-2400	2500-2600	2700-2800
Fruits	1.5-2 c.	1.5-2 c.	1.5-2 c.	2-2.5 c.	2-2.5 c.	2.5-3.5 c.	3.5-4.5 c.	3.5-4.5 c.
Vegetables	1.5-2 c.	2-2.5 c.	2.5-3 c.	2.5-3 c.	3-3.5 c.	3.5-4.5 c.	4.5-5 c.	4.5-5 c.
Grains	5 oz-eq.	5-6 oz-eq.	6-7 oz-eq.	6-7 oz-eq.	7-8 oz-eq.	8-9 oz-eq.	9-10 oz-eq.	10-11 oz-eq.
Meat & Beans	4 oz-eq.	5 oz-eq.	5-5.5 oz-eq.	5.5-6.5 oz-eq.	6.5-7 oz-eq.	7-7.5 oz-eq.	7-7.5 oz-eq.	7.5-8 oz-eq.
Milk	2-3 c.	3 c.	3 c.	3 c.	3 c.	3 c.	3 c.	3 c.
Healthy Oils	4 tsp.	5 tsp.	5 tsp.	6 tsp.	6 tsp.	7 tsp.	8 tsp.	8 tsp.

Day/Date:

Breakfast: _____ Lunch: _____

Dinner: _____ Snack: _____

Group	Fruits	Vegetables	Grains	Meat & Beans	Milk	Oils
Goal Amount						
Estimate Your Total						
Increase ⇧ or Decrease? ⇩						

Physical Activity: _____ Spiritual Activity: _____

Steps/Miles/Minutes: _____

Day/Date:

Breakfast: _____ Lunch: _____

Dinner: _____ Snack: _____

Group	Fruits	Vegetables	Grains	Meat & Beans	Milk	Oils
Goal Amount						
Estimate Your Total						
Increase ⇧ or Decrease? ⇩						

Physical Activity: _____ Spiritual Activity: _____

Steps/Miles/Minutes: _____

Day/Date:

Breakfast: _____ Lunch: _____

Dinner: _____ Snack: _____

Group	Fruits	Vegetables	Grains	Meat & Beans	Milk	Oils
Goal Amount						
Estimate Your Total						
Increase ⇧ or Decrease? ⇩						

Physical Activity: _____ Spiritual Activity: _____

Steps/Miles/Minutes: _____

Day/Date: _____

Breakfast: _____ Lunch: _____

Dinner: _____ Snack: _____

Group	Fruits	Vegetables	Grains	Meat & Beans	Milk	Oils
Goal Amount						
Estimate Your Total						
Increase ⇧ or Decrease? ⇩						

Physical Activity: _____ Spiritual Activity: _____

Steps/Miles/Minutes: _____

Day/Date: _____

Breakfast: _____ Lunch: _____

Dinner: _____ Snack: _____

Group	Fruits	Vegetables	Grains	Meat & Beans	Milk	Oils
Goal Amount						
Estimate Your Total						
Increase ⇧ or Decrease? ⇩						

Physical Activity: _____ Spiritual Activity: _____

Steps/Miles/Minutes: _____

Day/Date: _____

Breakfast: _____ Lunch: _____

Dinner: _____ Snack: _____

Group	Fruits	Vegetables	Grains	Meat & Beans	Milk	Oils
Goal Amount						
Estimate Your Total						
Increase ⇧ or Decrease? ⇩						

Physical Activity: _____ Spiritual Activity: _____

Steps/Miles/Minutes: _____

Day/Date: _____

Breakfast: _____ Lunch: _____

Dinner: _____ Snack: _____

Group	Fruits	Vegetables	Grains	Meat & Beans	Milk	Oils
Goal Amount						
Estimate Your Total						
Increase ⇧ or Decrease? ⇩						

Physical Activity: _____ Spiritual Activity: _____

Steps/Miles/Minutes: _____

Live It Tracker

Name: _____ Loss/gain: _____ lbs.

Date: _____ Week #: _____ Calorie Range: _____ My food goal for next week: _____

Activity Level: None, < 30 min/day, 30-60 min/day, 60+ min/day My activity goal for next week: _____

Group	Daily Calories							
	1300-1400	1500-1600	1700-1800	1900-2000	2100-2200	2300-2400	2500-2600	2700-2800
Fruits	1.5-2 c.	1.5-2 c.	1.5-2 c.	2-2.5 c.	2-2.5 c.	2.5-3.5 c.	3.5-4.5 c.	3.5-4.5 c.
Vegetables	1.5-2 c.	2-2.5 c.	2.5-3 c.	2.5-3 c.	3-3.5 c.	3.5-4.5 c.	4.5-5 c.	4.5-5 c.
Grains	5 oz-eq.	5-6 oz-eq.	6-7 oz-eq.	6-7 oz-eq.	7-8 oz-eq.	8-9 oz-eq.	9-10 oz-eq.	10-11 oz-eq.
Meat & Beans	4 oz-eq.	5 oz-eq.	5-5.5 oz-eq.	5.5-6.5 oz-eq.	6.5-7 oz-eq.	7-7.5 oz-eq.	7-7.5 oz-eq.	7.5-8 oz-eq.
Milk	2-3 c.	3 c.	3 c.	3 c.	3 c.	3 c.	3 c.	3 c.
Healthy Oils	4 tsp.	5 tsp.	5 tsp.	6 tsp.	6 tsp.	7 tsp.	8 tsp.	8 tsp.

Day/Date:

Breakfast: _____ Lunch: _____

Dinner: _____ Snack: _____

Group	Fruits	Vegetables	Grains	Meat & Beans	Milk	Oils
Goal Amount						
Estimate Your Total						
Increase ⇧ or Decrease? ⇩						

Physical Activity: _____ Spiritual Activity: _____

Steps/Miles/Minutes: _____ _____

Day/Date:

Breakfast: _____ Lunch: _____

Dinner: _____ Snack: _____

Group	Fruits	Vegetables	Grains	Meat & Beans	Milk	Oils
Goal Amount						
Estimate Your Total						
Increase ⇧ or Decrease? ⇩						

Physical Activity: _____ Spiritual Activity: _____

Steps/Miles/Minutes: _____ _____

Day/Date:

Breakfast: _____ Lunch: _____

Dinner: _____ Snack: _____

Group	Fruits	Vegetables	Grains	Meat & Beans	Milk	Oils
Goal Amount						
Estimate Your Total						
Increase ⇧ or Decrease? ⇩						

Physical Activity: _____ Spiritual Activity: _____

Steps/Miles/Minutes: _____ _____

Day/Date: ___

Breakfast: _____ Lunch: _____

Dinner: _____ Snack: _____

Group	Fruits	Vegetables	Grains	Meat & Beans	Milk	Oils
Goal Amount						
Estimate Your Total						
Increase ⇧ or Decrease? ⇩						

Physical Activity: _____ Spiritual Activity: _____

Steps/Miles/Minutes: _____ _____

Day/Date: ___

Breakfast: _____ Lunch: _____

Dinner: _____ Snack: _____

Group	Fruits	Vegetables	Grains	Meat & Beans	Milk	Oils
Goal Amount						
Estimate Your Total						
Increase ⇧ or Decrease? ⇩						

Physical Activity: _____ Spiritual Activity: _____

Steps/Miles/Minutes: _____ _____

Day/Date: ___

Breakfast: _____ Lunch: _____

Dinner: _____ Snack: _____

Group	Fruits	Vegetables	Grains	Meat & Beans	Milk	Oils
Goal Amount						
Estimate Your Total						
Increase ⇧ or Decrease? ⇩						

Physical Activity: _____ Spiritual Activity: _____

Steps/Miles/Minutes: _____ _____

Day/Date: ___

Breakfast: _____ Lunch: _____

Dinner: _____ Snack: _____

Group	Fruits	Vegetables	Grains	Meat & Beans	Milk	Oils
Goal Amount						
Estimate Your Total						
Increase ⇧ or Decrease? ⇩						

Physical Activity: _____ Spiritual Activity: _____

Steps/Miles/Minutes: _____ _____

Live It Tracker

Name: _____ Loss/gain: _____ lbs.

Date: _____ Week #: _____ Calorie Range: _____ My food goal for next week: _____

Activity Level: None, < 30 min/day, 30-60 min/day, 60+ min/day My activity goal for next week: _____

Group	Daily Calories							
	1300-1400	1500-1600	1700-1800	1900-2000	2100-2200	2300-2400	2500-2600	2700-2800
Fruits	1.5-2 c.	1.5-2 c.	1.5-2 c.	2-2.5 c.	2-2.5 c.	2.5-3.5 c.	3.5-4.5 c.	3.5-4.5 c.
Vegetables	1.5-2 c.	2-2.5 c.	2.5-3 c.	2.5-3 c.	3-3.5 c.	3.5-4.5 c.	4.5-5 c.	4.5-5 c.
Grains	5 oz-eq.	5-6 oz-eq.	6-7 oz-eq.	6-7 oz-eq.	7-8 oz-eq.	8-9 oz-eq.	9-10 oz-eq.	10-11 oz-eq.
Meat & Beans	4 oz-eq.	5 oz-eq.	5-5.5 oz-eq.	5.5-6.5 oz-eq.	6.5-7 oz-eq.	7-7.5 oz-eq.	7-7.5 oz-eq.	7.5-8 oz-eq.
Milk	2-3 c.	3 c.	3 c.	3 c.	3 c.	3 c.	3 c.	3 c.
Healthy Oils	4 tsp.	5 tsp.	5 tsp.	6 tsp.	6 tsp.	7 tsp.	8 tsp.	8 tsp.

Breakfast: _____ Lunch: _____

Dinner: _____ Snack: _____

Group	Fruits	Vegetables	Grains	Meat & Beans	Milk	Oils
Goal Amount						
Estimate Your Total						
Increase ⇧ or Decrease? ⇩						

Physical Activity: _____ Spiritual Activity: _____

Steps/Miles/Minutes: _____ _____

Breakfast: _____ Lunch: _____

Dinner: _____ Snack: _____

Group	Fruits	Vegetables	Grains	Meat & Beans	Milk	Oils
Goal Amount						
Estimate Your Total						
Increase ⇧ or Decrease? ⇩						

Physical Activity: _____ Spiritual Activity: _____

Steps/Miles/Minutes: _____ _____

Breakfast: _____ Lunch: _____

Dinner: _____ Snack: _____

Group	Fruits	Vegetables	Grains	Meat & Beans	Milk	Oils
Goal Amount						
Estimate Your Total						
Increase ⇧ or Decrease? ⇩						

Physical Activity: _____ Spiritual Activity: _____

Steps/Miles/Minutes: _____

Day/Date: _____

Breakfast: _____ Lunch: _____

Dinner: _____ Snack: _____

Group	Fruits	Vegetables	Grains	Meat & Beans	Milk	Oils
Goal Amount						
Estimate Your Total						
Increase ⇧ or Decrease? ⇩						

Physical Activity: _____ Spiritual Activity: _____

Steps/Miles/Minutes: _____ _____

Day/Date: _____

Breakfast: _____ Lunch: _____

Dinner: _____ Snack: _____

Group	Fruits	Vegetables	Grains	Meat & Beans	Milk	Oils
Goal Amount						
Estimate Your Total						
Increase ⇧ or Decrease? ⇩						

Physical Activity: _____ Spiritual Activity: _____

Steps/Miles/Minutes: _____ _____

Day/Date: _____

Breakfast: _____ Lunch: _____

Dinner: _____ Snack: _____

Group	Fruits	Vegetables	Grains	Meat & Beans	Milk	Oils
Goal Amount						
Estimate Your Total						
Increase ⇧ or Decrease? ⇩						

Physical Activity: _____ Spiritual Activity: _____

Steps/Miles/Minutes: _____ _____

Day/Date: _____

Breakfast: _____ Lunch: _____

Dinner: _____ Snack: _____

Group	Fruits	Vegetables	Grains	Meat & Beans	Milk	Oils
Goal Amount						
Estimate Your Total						
Increase ⇧ or Decrease? ⇩						

Physical Activity: _____ Spiritual Activity: _____

Steps/Miles/Minutes: _____ _____

Live It Tracker

Name: _____ Loss/gain: _____ lbs.

Date: _____ Week #: _____ Calorie Range: _____ My food goal for next week: _____

Activity Level: None, < 30 min/day, 30-60 min/day, 60+ min/day My activity goal for next week: _____

Group	Daily Calories							
	1300-1400	1500-1600	1700-1800	1900-2000	2100-2200	2300-2400	2500-2600	2700-2800
Fruits	1.5-2 c.	1.5-2 c.	1.5-2 c.	2-2.5 c.	2-2.5 c.	2.5-3.5 c.	3.5-4.5 c.	3.5-4.5 c.
Vegetables	1.5-2 c.	2-2.5 c.	2.5-3 c.	2.5-3 c.	3-3.5 c.	3.5-4.5 c.	4.5-5 c.	4.5-5 c.
Grains	5 oz-eq.	5-6 oz-eq.	6-7 oz-eq.	6-7 oz-eq.	7-8 oz-eq.	8-9 oz-eq.	9-10 oz-eq.	10-11 oz-eq.
Meat & Beans	4 oz-eq.	5 oz-eq.	5-5.5 oz-eq.	5.5-6.5 oz-eq.	6.5-7 oz-eq.	7-7.5 oz-eq.	7-7.5 oz-eq.	7.5-8 oz-eq.
Milk	2-3 c.	3 c.	3 c.	3 c.	3 c.	3 c.	3 c.	3 c.
Healthy Oils	4 tsp.	5 tsp.	5 tsp.	6 tsp.	6 tsp.	7 tsp.	8 tsp.	8 tsp.

Day/Date:

Breakfast: _____ Lunch: _____

Dinner: _____ Snack: _____

Group	Fruits	Vegetables	Grains	Meat & Beans	Milk	Oils
Goal Amount						
Estimate Your Total						
Increase ⇧ or Decrease? ⇩						

Physical Activity: _____ Spiritual Activity: _____

Steps/Miles/Minutes: _____

Day/Date:

Breakfast: _____ Lunch: _____

Dinner: _____ Snack: _____

Group	Fruits	Vegetables	Grains	Meat & Beans	Milk	Oils
Goal Amount						
Estimate Your Total						
Increase ⇧ or Decrease? ⇩						

Physical Activity: _____ Spiritual Activity: _____

Steps/Miles/Minutes: _____

Day/Date:

Breakfast: _____ Lunch: _____

Dinner: _____ Snack: _____

Group	Fruits	Vegetables	Grains	Meat & Beans	Milk	Oils
Goal Amount						
Estimate Your Total						
Increase ⇧ or Decrease? ⇩						

Physical Activity: _____ Spiritual Activity: _____

Steps/Miles/Minutes: _____

Day/Date: _____

Breakfast: _____ Lunch: _____

Dinner: _____ Snack: _____
_____ _____

Group	Fruits	Vegetables	Grains	Meat & Beans	Milk	Oils
Goal Amount						
Estimate Your Total						
Increase ⇧ or Decrease? ⇩						

Physical Activity: _____ Spiritual Activity: _____

Steps/Miles/Minutes: _____ _____

Day/Date: _____

Breakfast: _____ Lunch: _____

Dinner: _____ Snack: _____
_____ _____

Group	Fruits	Vegetables	Grains	Meat & Beans	Milk	Oils
Goal Amount						
Estimate Your Total						
Increase ⇧ or Decrease? ⇩						

Physical Activity: _____ Spiritual Activity: _____

Steps/Miles/Minutes: _____ _____

Day/Date: _____

Breakfast: _____ Lunch: _____

Dinner: _____ Snack: _____
_____ _____

Group	Fruits	Vegetables	Grains	Meat & Beans	Milk	Oils
Goal Amount						
Estimate Your Total						
Increase ⇧ or Decrease? ⇩						

Physical Activity: _____ Spiritual Activity: _____

Steps/Miles/Minutes: _____ _____

Day/Date: _____

Breakfast: _____ Lunch: _____

Dinner: _____ Snack: _____
_____ _____

Group	Fruits	Vegetables	Grains	Meat & Beans	Milk	Oils
Goal Amount						
Estimate Your Total						
Increase ⇧ or Decrease? ⇩						

Physical Activity: _____ Spiritual Activity: _____

Steps/Miles/Minutes: _____ _____

Live It Tracker

Name: _____ Loss/gain: _____ lbs.

Date: _____ Week #: ____ Calorie Range: _____ My food goal for next week: _____

Activity Level: None, < 30 min/day, 30-60 min/day, 60+ min/day My activity goal for next week: _____

Group	Daily Calories							
	1300-1400	1500-1600	1700-1800	1900-2000	2100-2200	2300-2400	2500-2600	2700-2800
Fruits	1.5-2 c.	1.5-2 c.	1.5-2 c.	2-2.5 c.	2-2.5 c.	2.5-3.5 c.	3.5-4.5 c.	3.5-4.5 c.
Vegetables	1.5-2 c.	2-2.5 c.	2.5-3 c.	2.5-3 c.	3-3.5 c.	3.5-4.5 c.	4.5-5 c.	4.5-5 c.
Grains	5 oz-eq.	5-6 oz-eq.	6-7 oz-eq.	6-7 oz-eq.	7-8 oz-eq.	8-9 oz-eq.	9-10 oz-eq.	10-11 oz-eq.
Meat & Beans	4 oz-eq.	5 oz-eq.	5-5.5 oz-eq.	5.5-6.5 oz-eq.	6.5-7 oz-eq.	7-7.5 oz-eq.	7-7.5 oz-eq.	7.5-8 oz-eq.
Milk	2-3 c.	3 c.	3 c.	3 c.	3 c.	3 c.	3 c.	3 c.
Healthy Oils	4 tsp.	5 tsp.	5 tsp.	6 tsp.	6 tsp.	7 tsp.	8 tsp.	8 tsp.

Day/Date:

Breakfast: _____ Lunch: _____

Dinner: _____ Snack: _____

Group	Fruits	Vegetables	Grains	Meat & Beans	Milk	Oils
Goal Amount						
Estimate Your Total						
Increase ⇧ or Decrease? ⇩						

Physical Activity: _____ Spiritual Activity: _____

Steps/Miles/Minutes: _____ _____

Day/Date:

Breakfast: _____ Lunch: _____

Dinner: _____ Snack: _____

Group	Fruits	Vegetables	Grains	Meat & Beans	Milk	Oils
Goal Amount						
Estimate Your Total						
Increase ⇧ or Decrease? ⇩						

Physical Activity: _____ Spiritual Activity: _____

Steps/Miles/Minutes: _____ _____

Day/Date:

Breakfast: _____ Lunch: _____

Dinner: _____ Snack: _____

Group	Fruits	Vegetables	Grains	Meat & Beans	Milk	Oils
Goal Amount						
Estimate Your Total						
Increase ⇧ or Decrease? ⇩						

Physical Activity: _____ Spiritual Activity: _____

Steps/Miles/Minutes: _____ _____

Day/Date: ______

Breakfast: ______

Lunch: ______

Dinner: ______

Snack: ______

Group	Fruits	Vegetables	Grains	Meat & Beans	Milk	Oils
Goal Amount						
Estimate Your Total						
Increase ⇧ or Decrease? ⇩						

Physical Activity: ______

Spiritual Activity: ______

Steps/Miles/Minutes: ______

Day/Date: ______

Breakfast: ______

Lunch: ______

Dinner: ______

Snack: ______

Group	Fruits	Vegetables	Grains	Meat & Beans	Milk	Oils
Goal Amount						
Estimate Your Total						
Increase ⇧ or Decrease? ⇩						

Physical Activity: ______

Spiritual Activity: ______

Steps/Miles/Minutes: ______

Day/Date: ______

Breakfast: ______

Lunch: ______

Dinner: ______

Snack: ______

Group	Fruits	Vegetables	Grains	Meat & Beans	Milk	Oils
Goal Amount						
Estimate Your Total						
Increase ⇧ or Decrease? ⇩						

Physical Activity: ______

Spiritual Activity: ______

Steps/Miles/Minutes: ______

Day/Date: ______

Breakfast: ______

Lunch: ______

Dinner: ______

Snack: ______

Group	Fruits	Vegetables	Grains	Meat & Beans	Milk	Oils
Goal Amount						
Estimate Your Total						
Increase ⇧ or Decrease? ⇩						

Physical Activity: ______

Spiritual Activity: ______

Steps/Miles/Minutes: ______

Live It Tracker

Name: _____ Loss/gain: _____ lbs.

Date: _____ Week #: _____ Calorie Range: _____ My food goal for next week: _____

Activity Level: None, < 30 min/day, 30-60 min/day, 60+ min/day My activity goal for next week: _____

Group	Daily Calories							
	1300-1400	1500-1600	1700-1800	1900-2000	2100-2200	2300-2400	2500-2600	2700-2800
Fruits	1.5-2 c.	1.5-2 c.	1.5-2 c.	2-2.5 c.	2-2.5 c.	2.5-3.5 c.	3.5-4.5 c.	3.5-4.5 c.
Vegetables	1.5-2 c.	2-2.5 c.	2.5-3 c.	2.5-3 c.	3-3.5 c.	3.5-4.5 c.	4.5-5 c.	4.5-5 c.
Grains	5 oz-eq.	5-6 oz-eq.	6-7 oz-eq.	6-7 oz-eq.	7-8 oz-eq.	8-9 oz-eq.	9-10 oz-eq.	10-11 oz-eq.
Meat & Beans	4 oz-eq.	5 oz-eq.	5-5.5 oz-eq.	5.5-6.5 oz-eq.	6.5-7 oz-eq.	7-7.5 oz-eq.	7-7.5 oz-eq.	7.5-8 oz-eq.
Milk	2-3 c.	3 c.	3 c.	3 c.	3 c.	3 c.	3 c.	3 c.
Healthy Oils	4 tsp.	5 tsp.	5 tsp.	6 tsp.	6 tsp.	7 tsp.	8 tsp.	8 tsp.

Day/Date: _____

Breakfast: _____ Lunch: _____

Dinner: _____ Snack: _____

Group	Fruits	Vegetables	Grains	Meat & Beans	Milk	Oils
Goal Amount						
Estimate Your Total						
Increase ⇧ or Decrease? ⇩						

Physical Activity: _____ Spiritual Activity: _____

Steps/Miles/Minutes: _____ _____

Day/Date: _____

Breakfast: _____ Lunch: _____

Dinner: _____ Snack: _____

Group	Fruits	Vegetables	Grains	Meat & Beans	Milk	Oils
Goal Amount						
Estimate Your Total						
Increase ⇧ or Decrease? ⇩						

Physical Activity: _____ Spiritual Activity: _____

Steps/Miles/Minutes: _____ _____

Day/Date: _____

Breakfast: _____ Lunch: _____

Dinner: _____ Snack: _____

Group	Fruits	Vegetables	Grains	Meat & Beans	Milk	Oils
Goal Amount						
Estimate Your Total						
Increase ⇧ or Decrease? ⇩						

Physical Activity: _____ Spiritual Activity: _____

Steps/Miles/Minutes: _____ _____

Day/Date:

Breakfast: _____ Lunch: _____

Dinner: _____ Snack: _____

Group	Fruits	Vegetables	Grains	Meat & Beans	Milk	Oils
Goal Amount						
Estimate Your Total						
Increase ⇧ or Decrease? ⇩						

Physical Activity: _____ Spiritual Activity: _____

Steps/Miles/Minutes: _____

Day/Date:

Breakfast: _____ Lunch: _____

Dinner: _____ Snack: _____

Group	Fruits	Vegetables	Grains	Meat & Beans	Milk	Oils
Goal Amount						
Estimate Your Total						
Increase ⇧ or Decrease? ⇩						

Physical Activity: _____ Spiritual Activity: _____

Steps/Miles/Minutes: _____

Day/Date:

Breakfast: _____ Lunch: _____

Dinner: _____ Snack: _____

Group	Fruits	Vegetables	Grains	Meat & Beans	Milk	Oils
Goal Amount						
Estimate Your Total						
Increase ⇧ or Decrease? ⇩						

Physical Activity: _____ Spiritual Activity: _____

Steps/Miles/Minutes: _____

Day/Date:

Breakfast: _____ Lunch: _____

Dinner: _____ Snack: _____

Group	Fruits	Vegetables	Grains	Meat & Beans	Milk	Oils
Goal Amount						
Estimate Your Total						
Increase ⇧ or Decrease? ⇩						

Physical Activity: _____ Spiritual Activity: _____

Steps/Miles/Minutes: _____

Live It Tracker

Name: _____ Loss/gain: _____ lbs.

Date: _____ Week #: _____ Calorie Range: _____ My food goal for next week: _____

Activity Level: None, < 30 min/day, 30-60 min/day, 60+ min/day My activity goal for next week: _____

Group	Daily Calories							
	1300-1400	1500-1600	1700-1800	1900-2000	2100-2200	2300-2400	2500-2600	2700-2800
Fruits	1.5-2 c.	1.5-2 c.	1.5-2 c.	2-2.5 c.	2-2.5 c.	2.5-3.5 c.	3.5-4.5 c.	3.5-4.5 c.
Vegetables	1.5-2 c.	2-2.5 c.	2.5-3 c.	2.5-3 c.	3-3.5 c.	3.5-4.5 c.	4.5-5 c.	4.5-5 c.
Grains	5 oz-eq.	5-6 oz-eq.	6-7 oz-eq.	6-7 oz-eq.	7-8 oz-eq.	8-9 oz-eq.	9-10 oz-eq.	10-11 oz-eq.
Meat & Beans	4 oz-eq.	5 oz-eq.	5-5.5 oz-eq.	5.5-6.5 oz-eq.	6.5-7 oz-eq.	7-7.5 oz-eq.	7-7.5 oz-eq.	7.5-8 oz-eq.
Milk	2-3 c.	3 c.	3 c.	3 c.	3 c.	3 c.	3 c.	3 c.
Healthy Oils	4 tsp.	5 tsp.	5 tsp.	6 tsp.	6 tsp.	7 tsp.	8 tsp.	8 tsp.

Day/Date:

Breakfast: _____ Lunch: _____

Dinner: _____ Snack: _____

Group	Fruits	Vegetables	Grains	Meat & Beans	Milk	Oils
Goal Amount						
Estimate Your Total						
Increase ⇧ or Decrease? ⇩						

Physical Activity: _____ Spiritual Activity: _____

Steps/Miles/Minutes: _____

Day/Date:

Breakfast: _____ Lunch: _____

Dinner: _____ Snack: _____

Group	Fruits	Vegetables	Grains	Meat & Beans	Milk	Oils
Goal Amount						
Estimate Your Total						
Increase ⇧ or Decrease? ⇩						

Physical Activity: _____ Spiritual Activity: _____

Steps/Miles/Minutes: _____

Day/Date:

Breakfast: _____ Lunch: _____

Dinner: _____ Snack: _____

Group	Fruits	Vegetables	Grains	Meat & Beans	Milk	Oils
Goal Amount						
Estimate Your Total						
Increase ⇧ or Decrease? ⇩						

Physical Activity: _____ Spiritual Activity: _____

Steps/Miles/Minutes: _____

Day/Date: _____

Breakfast: _____ Lunch: _____

Dinner: _____ Snack: _____

Group	Fruits	Vegetables	Grains	Meat & Beans	Milk	Oils
Goal Amount						
Estimate Your Total						
Increase ⇧ or Decrease? ⇩						

Physical Activity: _____ Spiritual Activity: _____

Steps/Miles/Minutes: _____ _____

Day/Date: _____

Breakfast: _____ Lunch: _____

Dinner: _____ Snack: _____

Group	Fruits	Vegetables	Grains	Meat & Beans	Milk	Oils
Goal Amount						
Estimate Your Total						
Increase ⇧ or Decrease? ⇩						

Physical Activity: _____ Spiritual Activity: _____

Steps/Miles/Minutes: _____ _____

Day/Date: _____

Breakfast: _____ Lunch: _____

Dinner: _____ Snack: _____

Group	Fruits	Vegetables	Grains	Meat & Beans	Milk	Oils
Goal Amount						
Estimate Your Total						
Increase ⇧ or Decrease? ⇩						

Physical Activity: _____ Spiritual Activity: _____

Steps/Miles/Minutes: _____ _____

Day/Date: _____

Breakfast: _____ Lunch: _____

Dinner: _____ Snack: _____

Group	Fruits	Vegetables	Grains	Meat & Beans	Milk	Oils
Goal Amount						
Estimate Your Total						
Increase ⇧ or Decrease? ⇩						

Physical Activity: _____ Spiritual Activity: _____

Steps/Miles/Minutes: _____ _____

let's count our miles!

Join the 100-Mile Club this Session

Can't walk that mile yet? Don't be discouraged! There are exercises you can do to strengthen your body and burn those extra calories. Keep a record on your Live It Tracker of the number of minutes you do these common physical activities, convert those minutes to miles following the chart below, and then mark off each mile you have completed on the chart found on the back of the back cover. Report your miles to your 100-Mile Club representative when you first arrive each week. Remember, you are not competing with anyone else . . . just yourself. Your job is to strive to reach 100 miles before the last meeting in this session. You can do it—just keep on moving!

Walking

slowly, 2 mph	30 min. = 156 cal. = 1 mile
moderately, 3 mph	20 min. = 156 cal. = 1 mile
very briskly, 4 mph	15 min. = 156 cal. = 1 mile
speed walking	10 min. = 156 cal. = 1 mile
up stairs	13 min. = 159 cal. = 1 mile

Running/Jogging

10 min. = 156 cal. = 1 mile

Cycling Outdoors

slowly, <10 mph	20 min. = 156 cal. = 1 mile
light effort, 10-12 mph	12 min. = 156 cal. = 1 mile
moderate effort, 12-14 mph	10 min. = 156 cal. = 1 mile
vigorous effort, 14-16 mph	7.5 min. = 156 cal. = 1 mile
very fast, 16-19 mph	6.5 min. = 152 cal. = 1 mile

Sports Activities

Playing tennis (singles)	10 min. = 156 cal. = 1 mile
Swimming	
light to moderate effort	11 min. = 152 cal. = 1 mile
fast, vigorous effort	7.5 min. = 156 cal. = 1 mile
Softball	15 min. = 156 cal. = 1 mile
Golf	20 min. = 156 cal = 1 mile
Rollerblading	6.5 min. = 152 cal. = 1 mile
Ice skating	11 min. = 152 cal. = 1 mile

Jumping rope	7.5 min. = 156 cal. = 1 mile
Basketball	12 min. = 156 cal. = 1 mile
Soccer (casual)	15 min. = 159 cal. = 1 mile

Around the House

Mowing grass	22 min. = 156 cal. = 1 mile
Mopping, sweeping, vacuuming	19.5 min. = 155 cal. = 1 mile
Cooking	40 min. =160 cal. = 1 mile
Gardening	19 min. = 156 cal. = 1 mile
Housework (general)	35 min. = 156 cal. = 1 mile
Ironing	45 min. = 153 cal. = 1 mile
Raking leaves	25 min. = 150 cal. = 1 mile
Washing car	23 min. = 156 cal. = 1 mile
Washing dishes	45 min. = 153 cal. = 1 mile

At the Gym

Stair machine	8.5 min. = 155 cal. = 1 mile
Stationary bike	
slowly, 10 mph	30 min. = 156 cal. = 1 mile
moderately, 10-13 mph	15 min. = 156 cal. = 1 mile
vigorously, 13-16 mph	7.5 min. = 156 cal. = 1 mile
briskly, 16-19 mph	6.5 min. = 156 cal. = 1 mile
Elliptical trainer	12 min. = 156 cal. = 1 mile
Weight machines (used vigorously)	13 min. = 152 cal.=1 mile
Aerobics	
low impact	15 min. = 156 cal. = 1 mile
high impact	12 min. = 156 cal. = 1 mile
water	20 min. = 156 cal. = 1 mile
Pilates	15 min. = 156 cal. = 1 mile
Raquetball (casual)	15 min. = 159 cal. = 1 mile
Stretching exercises	25 min. = 150 cal. = 1 mile
Weight lifting (also works for weight machines used moderately or gently)	30 min. = 156 cal. = 1 mile

Family Leisure

Playing piano	37 min. = 155 cal. = 1 mile
Jumping rope	10 min. = 152 cal. = 1 mile
Skating (moderate)	20 min. = 152 cal. = 1 mile
Swimming	
moderate	17 min. = 156 cal. = 1 mile
vigorous	10 min. = 148 cal. = 1 mile
Table tennis	25 min. = 150 cal. = 1 mile
Walk/run/play with kids	25 min. = 150 cal. = 1 mile

Week 2: Making a Fresh Start

Therefore, if anyone is in Christ, he is a new creation; the old has gone, the new has come!

Week 3: Learning from the Past

And we know that in all things God works for the good of those who love him, who have been called according to his purpose.

A New Beginning

A New Beginning
Scripture Memory Verses:

2 CORINTHIANS 5:17   COLOSSIANS 3:23
  ROMANS 8:28   JOHN 1:16
    MICAH 6:8   PHILIPPIANS 2:10-11
2 CORINTHIANS 12:9   JOSHUA 1:5
  PHILIPPIANS 1:6   ISAIAH 40:31

HOW TO USE THESE CARDS:

Separate cards from the Bible study book. These cards are designed to be used when exercising. To do this, you may want to punch a hole in the upper left corner of the cards and place on a ring. When you have finished memorizing all the verses from one study, add the new Bible study cards to the ring and continue practicing the old verses while learning the new ones. Cards may be placed anywhere you will see them regularly—on the dashboard of your car, on a mirror, on a desk. After you have memorized the verse, begin using the reverse side of the card so the reference is connected to the verse. This is a great way to practice the verses you have already learned.

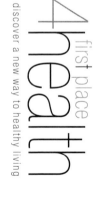

first place 4health

discover a new way to healthy living

2 CORINTHIANS 5:17

ROMANS 8:28

Week 6: Looking Ahead

Being confident of this, that he who began a good work in you will carry it on to completion until the day of Christ Jesus.

Week 7: Giving Our Best

Whatever you do, work at it with all your heart, as working for the Lord, not for men.

Week 4: Living in the Present

He has showed you, O man, what is good. And what does the LORD require of you? To act justly and to love mercy and to walk humbly with your God.

Week 5: Leaning on Jesus

But he said to me, "My grace is sufficient for you, for my power is made perfect in weakness." Therefore I will boast all the more gladly about my weaknesses, so that Christ's power may rest on me.

PHILIPPIANS 1:6

MICAH 6:8

COLOSSIANS 3:23

2 CORINTHIANS 12:9

Week 10: Standing by Faith

No one will be able to stand up against you all the days of your life. As I was with Moses, so I will be with you; I will never leave you nor forsake you.

Week 11: Soaring in the Strength of the Spirit

But those who hope in the LORD will renew their strength. They will soar on wings like eagles; they will run and not grow weary, they will walk and not be faint.

Week 8: Growing in Grace

From the fullness of his grace we have all received one blessing after another.

Week 9: Surrendering to His Lordship

That at the name of Jesus every knee should bow, in heaven and on earth and under the earth, and every tongue confess that Jesus Christ is Lord, to the glory of God the Father.

JOSHUA 1:5

JOHN 1:16

ISAIAH 40:31

PHILIPPIANS 2:10-11